VOLUME TWO

HEALTH PLANNING IN THE UNITED STATES:

Selected Policy Issues

Committee on Health Planning Goals and Standards

Institute of Medicine

NATIONAL ACADEMY PRESS
Washington, D.C.   1981

NOTICE The project that is the subject of this report
was approved by the Governing Board of the National Research Council, whose members are drawn from the Councils
of the National Academy of Sciences, the National Academy
of Engineering, and the Institute of Medicine. The members of the committee responsible for the report were
chosen for their special competencies and with regard
for appropriate balance.
    This report has been reviewed by a group other than
the authors according to procedures approved by a Report
Review Committee consisting of members of the National
Academy of Sciences, the National Academy of Engineering,
and the Institute of Medicine.

The Institute of Medicine was chartered in 1970 by the
National Academy of Sciences to enlist distinguished members of the appropriate professions in the examination of
policy matters pertaining to the health of the public.
In this, the Institute acts under both the Academy's
1863 Congressional charter responsibility to be an ad-
visor to the Federal Government, and its own initiative
in identifying issues of medical care, research, and
education.

Supported by the Health Resources Administration Contract
No. 282-78-0163-EJM

LIBRARY OF CONGRESS CATALOGING IN PUBLICATION DATA

National Academy of Sciences (U.S.). Institute of
    Medicine. Committee on Health Planning Goals
    and Standards.
    Health planning in the United States.

    Bibliography: v. 2, p.
    1. Health planning—United States. 2. Medical
policy—United States. I. Title. [DNLM: 1. Health
planning—United States. WA 540 AA1 H227]
RA395.A3N285 1981   362.1'06   81-9534
ISBN 0-309-03145-1 (v. 2)   AACR2

Available from:

National Academy Press
2101 Constitution Ave., N.W.
Washington, D.C. 20418

Printed in the United States of America

COMMITTEE ON HEALTH PLANNING
GOALS AND STANDARDS

LIAISON MEMBERS FROM THE NATIONAL COUNCIL ON HEALTH
PLANNING AND DEVELOPMENT:

S. PHILIP CAPER, Vice Chancellor for Health Affairs and
   Professor of Medicine, University of Massachusetts
   Medical Center
L. EMMERSON WARD, Professor of Medicine, Mayo Medical
   School

PREFACE

This volume is composed of the background papers commissioned by a committee of the Institute of Medicine. The committee was formed to study health planning in the United States. A list of the committee's members, including its chairman, Rashi Fein, Ph.D., is provided at the front of this volume. The papers in this volume detail the empirical and theoretical underpinnings of the second year's report, which discusses national, state, and local relationships and consumer participation in health planning. The authors in this volume were encouraged to express their opinions and make their own recommendations. The papers, although reviewed by the Academy, are not submitted to the same review process as committee reports and represent the views of the individual authors, not the committee or the Institute of Medicine. The committee feels that the papers by themselves constitute major contributions to the quality of current debates in health planning and should be disseminated broadly.

Helen Darling
Study Director

CONTENTS

vii

SOME STRUCTURAL ISSUES
IN THE HEALTH PLANNING PROGRAM

Lawrence D. Brown

*Health Systems Agencies (HSAs) were established by P.L.
93-641 as the mechanism of local health planning. In
this paper Brown describes the structure and internal
organization of HSAs, their relationships with the organizations with which they must interact, and the
political forces with which they must contend. Brown
highlights many issues that inhibit the effective working
of the HSAs, and concludes with some suggestions for
reforms that might improve the contribution of HSAs to
the health planning effort.*

"We designed it backwards."--Official in the U.S.
Department of Health and Human Services.

That planning is inseparable from politics is a truism.
The corollary--that planning is therefore also inseparable
from political structure--is less familiar.[1] Political
"structures"--the explicit distribution of roles and
powers among official participants in a public program
and the informal distribution that both official and
unofficial participants invent to supplement these explicit arrangements--do much to define the rules of the
policy game and the balance of power among interests.
   A new federal program raises three central structural
questions: first, How will the program be organized in-
ternally? ("organizational" questions); second, How will
it fit with existing programs in its immediate (usually
state or local) environment? ("environmental" questions);
and third, What requirements, regulations, and informal
understandings will bind it to its federal creators and

1

administrators? ("federal" questions). These questions
are especially important when the federal government
tries to meet its objectives by creating and working
through a new organization--for example, the Health
Systems Agencies (HSAs) with which this paper deals.
An organization-building effort is not content to alter
existing organizational and intergovernmental arrangements at the margin, as by means of new requirements
and incentives attached to grants-in-aid. Instead it
injects a new organizational presence--a new structure--
into the existing set of programs. Building a new organization is more complicated than deciding what conditions to attach to grants-in-aid. Fitting a new organization into the universe of state and local organizations
is more complex than trying to alter the behavior of
some member of that universe in delimited respects.
Trying to decide how the trade-off between federal control and local autonomy affects the capacities of a new
organization is more difficult than attempting to assert
"the influence of federal grants"[2] incrementally over
time in established programs.

These structural questions are highly pertinent in
the health planning field, where organization-building has
been central to the federal government's strategy.[3] In
1974, convinced that the nation needed a network of area
and state-based health planning bodies, but that the
Comprehensive Health Planning (CHP) agencies created in
1966 had proved to be too weak, the federal government
set out to strengthen the CHP model. The health planning
bodies established in the Health Planning and Resources
Development Act of 1974 (P.L. 93-641) were to be known as
Health Systems Agencies. In each state one or more HSAs
would assume responsibility for drawing up long-term
"health systems plans" (HSPs) and "annual implementation
plans" (AIPs) that considered the needs of their jurisdiction and the degree to which present and projected resources and resource development patterns were adequate,
excessive, or insufficient. The agency itself would be
run by a governing board, the structure of which was set
forth in considerable detail. It was to be composed of
representatives of consumers, providers, local organizations, and special income, racial, linguistic, and other
groups. Consumers were required to constitute a majority
of the board. As of November 1979, there were 202 HSAs,
16 of which crossed state lines and 12 of which covered
an entire state.[4]

The law also prescribed new intergovernmental arrangements. To assure coordination and planning on the proper scale, it required that the work of the HSAs be coordinated by a single state agency, the so-called State Health Planning and Development Agency (SHPDA), which would synthesize HSA plans into a statewide plan subject in turn to the approval of a Statewide Health Coordinating Council (SHCC), a majority of whose members would come from HSAs within the state. The plans would be considered by federal grant-giving agencies in the review of applications for funds (so-called "proposed use of federal funds" or PUFF reviews) and by the states in their reviews of applications by health care institutions for "certificates of need" (CON). These state and local bodies are themselves subject to regulations and guidelines issued by the Department of Health and Human Services (DHHS) (until recently called the Department of Health, Education, and Welfare), advised by a National Council on Health Planning and Resources Development.

Thus, the federal government has chosen to strengthen health planning in the United States by establishing new local--and state and federal--organizations and by conferring on them significant planning responsibilities and regulatory powers. These powers, located along the hazy line between review and comment and review and sign-off, are rather weak regulatory weapons. Yet the powers, and still more the presence, of the HSAs, SHPDAs, and SHCCs are of considerable political importance. The official expression of a federally created "voice of the people" on health planning questions can legitimatize or impugn professional, institutional, and "grassroots" initiatives and can thereby help shape the nature of health care debates and perhaps even tip the balance of power in state and local health politics decisively to one or another side.

This paper, which summarizes impressions drawn from the author's research in progress on the implementation of health planning and regulatory efforts in Maryland, Washington, Michigan, and New York states, addresses the question whether the structural arrangements adopted by the federal government for health planning are adequate to the ambitious goals set for the planning process. In evaluating the structure of such a program, level of detail is not a sure indicator of level of sophistication. Program designers may address structural questions in minute detail and still miss the most important ones.

Details may stem from a realistic and dispassionate understanding of institutional patterns "out there," or they may reflect the designers' ideologies, certain intuitively or widely held prejudices about "how things work," or the need to smooth rough legislative edges to win the support or assuage the opposition of important groups.

As Raab's paper in this volume demonstrates,[5] the structure of the planning system strongly reflected the values and world view of its designers, especially of the congressional staffs who developed the legislation in detail. This outlook took a dim view of the contribution of state and local politicians and administrators to health planning: their parochialism, susceptibility to interest group influence, and general inefficiencies, it was thought, made it highly desirable to limit their planning roles.[6] Thus, in most cases, the HSAs were to be not public but private, nonprofit agencies. But if the designers disdained conventional politics, they valued pluralism highly. They recognized that providers, consumers, and other community interests must be involved in plan development and viewed the HSA as a suitable forum for working out their differences precisely *because* it was a new and self-contained organization, at arms length from the "pols" and civil servants. Even so the "partisan mutual adjustment"[7] of interest group interaction was not what the designers had in mind: the planning process was to be rigorous, technocratic, and rational.[8] Presumably these qualities were thought to follow from the emphasis the designers placed on "checks and balances," on fashioning a structure that would withstand the dominance of politician, bureaucrat, and professional alike, and indeed of any single special interest. Agencies endowed with the countervailing power of a consumer majority and an admixture of various community "factions" would arrive at a reasonable and efficient understanding of the community's true interest and then embody it in plans.

There is room for disagreement over whether this blend of antipolitical animus, pluralism, technocracy, and countervailing power was a coup of theoretical ingenuity or a fatuously inplausible construct. It is beyond doubt, however, that the cohesion of this precarious assemblage of values and processes depends heavily on the structure of the HSA and its related institutions. If for some reason the HSA organizations fail to work as intended,

the premises of the program cannot be maintained and
the expected conclusions do not follow. It is useful
therefore to turn to the three structural questions mentioned at the start of this paper--organizational,
environmental, and federal--and examine the realism of
the designers' work.

THE HSA AS AN ORGANIZATION

Examination of the organizational structure of the HSAs
usually, and properly, begins with analysis of the HSA
board. In 1977, for example, Bruce Vladeck persuasively
argued that the HSA strategy and structure are in many
ways at odds. Assembling around a table representatives
of a wide range of local interests is not likely to produce the dispassionate and rational planning modeled in
the texts. Instead it creates a highly politicized body
in which the surest road to consensus is the splitting of
particularistic and parochial differences by means of
bargaining, logrolling, and pork barreling.[9]

HSA's behavior cannot be entirely predicted from the
composition of their governing boards, however, for these
boards are but the tip of an organizational iceberg. The
boards consist of part-time "volunteers" meeting intermittently to consider proposals developed in other settings. These other settings--the work units of the
organization--deserve attention in their own right.
First, however, it is necessary to consider the nature
of the HSA's work.

The HSA's mandated mission is broad, complex, and
ambiguous. According to one account, "The agency's
primary responsibility is the provision of effective
health planning for its area and the promotion of the
development (within the area) of health services, manpower, and facilities which meet identified needs, reduce documented inefficiencies and implement the health
plans of the agency."[10] This definition emphasizes
"planning" and "promotion." Yet the same account implies
that the heart of the HSA's mission may be mainly research. For example: "The Plans must . . . describe
and characterize the status of the entire health system,
noting the effects that changes in one part of the system
may have on other parts. . . ." They must emphasize "a
systemwide approach with specified, quantified goals,
and the addition of information on costs and financing

(and the effects of proposed goals on cost containment
goals). . . . Moreover, "the agency must consider the
array of influences on health. In developing their
plans . . . agencies are expected to identify all relevant health factors and problems . . . and where possible
isolate those conditions which can be addressed by the
delivery system. . . ."[11]

In practice, however, it appears that a fourth mission
may be most important: cost containment by means of
regulation of capital investment. A recent study of
health planning in New England found that most of the
agencies studied "accept regulation as their first
priority. . . ."[12] And Basil Mott writes that "cost
containment is the driving force behind P.L. 93-641."[13]

There appear, then, to be at least four distinct
components to the HSA mission: research, planning, regulation, and advocacy (promotion). Unfortunately,
organizational arrangements suitable for one of these
tasks may not be suitable for others. For example, the
very systematic and ambitious research described above
will require the skills of highly trained academic experts and will take years. Planning presupposes an
adequate research base to support the plans, but requires
a rather different mix of skills: not the ability to do
research but rather the capacity to understand it and to
apply it intelligently and flexibly to the specifics of
a local situation. Regulation calls for a high degree of
legal and political skill for it entails the application
of a plan to institutions and the defense of those
applications against the laments (and suits) of aggrieved
interests. Advocacy, finally, requires a talent for reducing complex matters to readily understandable terms,
the rhetorical power to stir the blood, and the organizational ability to mobilize some community interests for
and against others. It is difficult to picture one agency
performing well all four tasks simultaneously.

Given the breadth, diversity, and complexity of the
HSA missions, it is not surprising that participants sometimes express uncertainty over the nature of the enterprise
on which they have embarked. As the executive director
of an HSA in Washington State put it in an interview:
"A basic underlying problem is, it's sort of like building
a ship. It's a big enterprise. You have to put all the
parts together. But it's not been decided what kind of
ship it's going to be, or even if it's going to be a
ship, or what it's evolving toward." Some even appear to

doubt whether the HSAs are principally health agencies at all. Thus, Checkoway cites one director who describes the HSA as a "social planning agency focusing on health" and another who views it as "an agency for social change."[14]

A rationally designed program would presumably begin by deciding the "outputs" it wishes to achieve, would then prescribe "processes" (activities) that conduce toward those ends, and would finally define the "inputs" (personnel and other resources) needed to sustain those processes. The intended outputs of the planning process may be interpreted to be anything from cost containment to social change, with many ambiguous possibilities in between. The prescribed processes encompass research, planning, regulation, and advocacy. And it is questionable that the participatory, corporative structure of the HSAs is well suited to support any, let alone all, of these processes.

Because each of the various ends and activities has influential proponents, HSAs must attempt in practice to honor all of them. In essence, the HSA mission is to assemble a representative and committee subset of community volunteers and then bring these members together to canvass rigorously and scientifically virtually the entire range of health needs and resources in the community, "compare" (in some sense) needs with resources, devise a long-range plan that rationally relates needs to resources, and then rework the long-term plan into a short-term plan of sufficient clarity and specificity that it may serve as a defensible basis for making detailed decisions about resources and services in the area in the present and future. It need hardly be said that these are not easy tasks. No one knows how to make these judgments "in general." Although various planning methodologies may be culled from the literature, none is self-evidently correct, and partisans dispute hotly about the merits of different approaches.[15] The problem is aggravated by the HSA structure, which transforms the agency's environment into organizational participants. HSA board members meet collectively only on occasion and many may be only casually interested in a matter at hand. But that matter may be of intense and immediate concern to a subset of board members or to well-connected executives of local health care organizations. Therefore, if the HSA is to go beyond the formulation of bland and nonspecific plans, it must be prepared to fight--within its own ranks and in the community--for the stand it takes.

The central organizational problem of the HSAs is how
to make their herculean tasks--"near impossible" of
attainment[16]--more nearly manageable. Their response is
the age-old expedient of division of labor; that is, they
divide their members and staff into subgroups and ask
them to specialize in portions of the tasks at hand.
Division of labor in HSAs takes three main forms: committees, staff, and subarea councils (SACs). The heart
of HSA decision-making is to be found in these three
subunits. But these subunits, vital as they are to the
organization's workings, also act as centrifugal forces,
pulling control away from the center (the executive
director and the board) and fragmenting the agency's
identity and unity of viewpoint. HSA management is
therefore a constant and sometimes hopeless struggle to
reconcile the virtues of comprehensive planning with the
virtues of decentralized work groups.

Committees

Like other organizations facing complex tasks, the HSA's
first and basic response to complexity is to break up and
farm it out. Thus, an HSA usually divides its board
members into a half-dozen or more subject-matter committees, each comprised of roughly 5 to 10 members, roughly
half consumer and half provider.[17] Committees tend to
be of four general types: (1) administration--personnel,
budget, and so on, of which no further account will be
taken here; (2) "need assessment"--primary care, mental
health, prevention, and the like (these committees concentrate on documenting and advancing neglected needs
and services); (3) regulatory--especially facilities and
grant review; and (4) plan development--drawing up the
long- and short-term plans on which HSA decisions are expected to rest, or at any rate, with which they are supposed to be consistent. The committees institutionalize
within the agency a split personality. Need assessment
committees make it their business to act as spokesmen for
more and new services. Regulatory committees are asked to
make constraining decisions that require trimming fat and
arguing for "less." There is no logical reason why the
two tasks must conflict, why denying new acute care beds
to a hospital must complicate assessment of the need for
a new outpatient clinic. In many cases complications do

arise, however. One reason is that meeting needs may require new grant funds or new facilities. Another is that hospitals themselves may suggest such compromises as expansion of outpatient services in exchange for a favorable HSA recommendation on a bed expansion, modernization project, or new piece of equipment. In these cases, relations between the need assessment and regulatory committees can become confused or conflictual, and the plan development committees, expected to produce a document that both saves money and does justice to the community's real (including its "unmet") needs, may get caught in the cross fire.

Aggregating committee positions into a united agency stand is further complicated by the need for plan development committees to assume a holistic, "systemwide" perspective, while the need assessment and regulatory committees adopt what might be termed an "institutional" orientation. Their decisions turn on such questions as whether institution X is doing all it could for (say) the cause of health education, whether it has demonstrated that the community needs its proposed construction or modernization project, and so forth.

Staff

Because their members are part-time volunteers and their tasks are very broad and complex, HSAs depend heavily on full-time staff. Yet, staff recruitment is often more difficult than recruiting members of the board. HSAs are new bodies, with uncertain futures, sometimes in fairly remote locations, therefore offering uncertain career prospects, and relatively low salaries. None of this necessarily bothers board members who have volunteered their interest in health planning, call their communities their home, participate "on the side," and do not get paid. All of it, however, may trouble staffers who wish to advance their careers, may be compelled to relocate families, will work for the HSA full-time, and must make a decent living. For these reasons, an HSA staff position is likely to be attractive mainly to young men and women with master's degrees in health planning or administration (or related fields), often hesitating between a personal or ideological commitment to planning and public service, and the practical advantages of a university doctoral program, a job in the private sector, or a civil service career. Staff, then, are "plan-oriented"; they are offered an HSA job because they are thought to command the "how to do it" methodological skills of which planning is thought to consist, and they accept such an offer because they are eager to practice their planning skills in the public interest (at least for a time).[18]

Staff are indispensable, but integrating a corps of planning experts into a multifactional, lay-dominated HSA poses problems. First, suitable staff are difficult to recruit and retain. For several reasons--clashes with the agency's director, isolated location of the agency, low salaries, and heavy workloads, for example[19]--high staff turnover has been a problem for many HSAs. Turnover means not only the loss of manpower, but also in many cases the loss of the one or few persons who truly understood (or claimed to understand) the arcane assumptions and quantitative methods that support the plan. When the staffer who patiently and at length managed to persuade the members of the facilities review committee and then the HSA board as a whole that the "Walsh-Bicknell" approach is the one true method of evaluating certificate of need applications departs and is replaced by a colleague with severe reservations about Walsh-Bicknell but full confidence in a rival method, the ensuing "reorienting and training and a new approach to the planning process"[20] may leave consumers and providers alike glassy-eyed and disgusted.

Even if staff tenure is long, however, the danger that the laymen will feel taken in or otherwise ill-served by staff remains. Staff tend to make an odd mix with local consumers and medical professionals on the board and in committees, most of whom know a lot about their communities and institutions and little about the formalities of planning. Whereas board and committee members are apt to emphasize the particular needs, roles, and failings of particular institutions, staff tend to concentrate on the proper role of one institution in the context of others, that is, in the overall plan. Volunteers may then consider the staff to be unduly rigid and may fear that they are being pushed or backed by staff into positions they do not really want to endorse. In the words of the Consumer Coalition for Health:[21]

> Many participants in the planning process, consumer and provider alike, complain about staff control of information, deadlines, etc. Staff *rarely* are

willing to present controversial alternatives to
planning decisions, i.e., analyses of the actual
effectiveness of medical technology being pur-
chased, expanded options as to how money might
best be used, etc.
. . . Consumers rarely become interested in
health planning *per se*. They become interested
because of specific issues: access, barriers,
quality, costs. HSA staff rarely help consumers
learn how to use the HSA's powers to solve these
problems. Instead, the consumers are led a merry
chase through HSPs, AIPs, square footage formulae,
and debt ratios, etc. Small wonder that there are
so many drop-outs.

The staff skills required in an HSA are more than
merely methodological. Politically sophisticated staff,
of whom there are many, work closely with consumer members of the HSA to resist "provider dominance" and help
pull the agency together in defense of stands unpopular
in the community. Not all staff are politically adept,
however, and even those who are may find managing the
many conflicts that arise in the HSA's complex intra-
and interorganizational milieu--conflicts within and between committees, within and between consumer and provider factions, and within and between the HSA "as a
whole" and the community, for example--to be an exhausting
and perhaps impossible job.

Subarea Councils

Many of the HSAs are built on the geographical, organizational, and personal foundations of the older CHPs, and
many--by one count 105 of the 205 HSA areas[22]--retain
the subarea councils to which CHP planning was often
delegated. Local area-oriented activitists who have
become accustomed to speaking for the needs of their
communities may be reluctant to blend their voice with
that of a new regional HSA presence, that is, a central
office executive director, board, and staff. Because
subarea councils are often the source of nominations
for positions on the HSA board, the subareas may be the
board members' principal constituencies, which may in
turn make the board members solicitous of subarea
autonomy.

One West Coast HSA, for example, tried to resolve
these tensions by describing itself as a "federation."
Soon, impressed by experience and by federal complaints
that a loose assemblage of warmed-over subarea documents
was not "planning," it resolved to avoid the term "federation" and to build a strong central capacity to assert
a systemwide perspective. (Its success to date has been
very limited.) These tensions can be severe when SACs
and HSA facilities review committees clash over who is to
be the agency's true spokesman for local certificate of
need reviews. They are most severe when an expansion-
minded rural underserved SAC meets skeptical reaction to
a certificate of need it favors in a regional facilities
review committee. According to a study of the HSAs in
federal Region X, which includes the states of Alaska,
Washington, Oregon, and Idaho, even in agencies where the
SACs do not dominate the HSA, "these bodies are exercising
a great deal of influence on the review process. HSAs
appear to be extremely sensitive to pressure from their
sub-areas."[23]

The central management task of HSA leadership is
neither comprehensive planning nor negotiating agreements
among members of the HSA board; rather it is developing
and staffing this three-part organizational structure
and then reconciling the distinctive contributions of
these subunits--institution-oriented committees, plan-
oriented staff, and area-oriented subarea councils. The
complexity of organization-building takes a great deal of
time--time ironically diverted from the planning enterprise. Almost 5 years after passage of the planning law,
a survey of Region X HSAs found that ". . . most of the
agencies have been more concerned with internal problems
and meeting designation deadlines than with their relationships to the external environment."[24] As a result, plans
have often been rushed and superficial. HEW-HHS delays
in issuing regulations and guidelines addressing these
internal questions are partly to blame. But one should
not infer from this that more time and guidance will make
the plans deliberative and profound. As these organizational structures become articulated, entrenched, and
committed, tensions and clashes of viewpoint may become
more frequent. The management task is largely one of
negotiating and keeping peace among internal subunits.
The plan is largely a "resultant" of internal organizational politics.

13

THE HSA IN ITS STATE AND LOCAL ENVIRONMENT

A second structural question about health planning concerns the HSA's ability to exert *inter*organizational influence, that is, its success in getting its work (plan, decision, advice, whatever) taken seriously by other organizations in the health care field at the local and state levels. The United States has never looked favorably on master or central planning bodies with strong powers. Therefore, planners are often charged with developing a plan the precise uses of which in shaping the larger world of public policy tend to be ambiguous. The influence of planning agencies tends to lie not in clear lines of authority but in interorganizational networks of persuasion and interest. The HSAs are no exception. As one federal official put it: "The annual implementation plan must be the *community's* workplan. The HSA by itself can't do a damn thing."

In theory, HSAs should be of major interest to other health regulatory bodies. For example, HSA "appropriateness" reviews and data and analyses about the institutional needs of an area might help the Professional Standards Review Organizations (PSROs) put their norms in context. Instead of simply assuming that prevailing practice patterns are right and proper, an HSA/PSRO dialogue would ask whether these patterns are in fact appropriate under alternative institutional assumptions-- for example, fewer beds here or an ambulatory surgical center there. These are questions the PSROs themselves tend not to pursue.

Again, certificate-of-need staff in the SHPDAs might be expected to depend heavily on HSA deliberations on the need for hospitals and other institutional alternatives, for CON staffs are often too few and too burdened with the details of particular cases to take a broad and synoptic view of community needs. The same may be said of state rate-setters, who typically examine individual hospital budgets or categories of budgets and have neither the time nor the mandate to address broad questions about the community's needs for various types and mixes of services. In all these areas the "big picture" supplied by HSAs should fill important gaps and give more narrowly focused regulators greater insight into the roots and ramifications of their work. In practice, however, HSAs have not yet exerted much influence on these agencies. There are several reasons.

HSA Difficulties

It is to be expected that the demand for the HSAs' prod-
ucts will bear some relation to the perceived quality
and usefulness of what the HSAs supply. However, for
reasons set out above--in particular, the strains of
establishing and then running a generalist organization
that must specialize sufficiently to address a very
broad, diverse, and complex mission--many HSAs remain
mired in their own formation and maintenance problems
and have therefore been unable to produce careful, useful, and pointed plans. The quality of plans differs
from place to place, but few would deny that some HSA
plans are little more than laundry lists of projects,
wish lists of general "priorities" and "emphases," or
compendia of updated CHP planning exercises. Frequently
the plans do not achieve a level of specificity that
carries clear implications for the daily tasks of more
focused regulators, and even when they do, these regulators (for example, PSROs, SHPDA staff, and hospital
rate-setters) often have methods and ideas of their
own, quite different from those of the HSA.

Organizational Definitions of Role and Mission

PSROs have had little use (at least to date) for HSA
thoughts on the relationship between institutional needs
and local norms governing hospital use. Most of the
reasons derive from the different ways in which the
organizations define (in Selznick's term) their "distinctive competence."[25] For one thing, most of the questions
of central interest to the HSAs fall outside the basic
PSRO mandate, which is not to speculate about systems-
change but rather to monitor the care of patients covered
by certain federal programs. Moreover, the PSROs view
themselves as professional peer groups monitoring, educa-
ting, and disciplining peers; their workings are an
intraprofessional affair and publicity is abhorrent to
them. The HSAs, by contrast, are multiconstituency bodies
that pride themselves on openness, participation, and
publicity. PSROs have therefore been unwilling to release
to HSAs--or to other onlookers--information naming particular hospitals, doctors, and patients. Even apart from
their "duty" of confidentiality, PSROs view themselves as
an elite with a monopoly on the interpretation of the

medical information they gather. One observer summarized their view as follows: "Even if PSRO data went to HSAs, who'd know how to use them? Very few. It's a slow process of education. Having unskilled, undiplomatic planners using complex data about providers for their own purposes is not necessarily in the public interest." In sum, the HSAs and PSROs have very different organizational characters--the one a broad-gauged planning body, the other a highly focused monitoring body; the one a public, participatory forum, the other a mode of professional self-regulation--and these distinctions set limits on the degree of coordination they seek.

Relations between state rate-setting agencies and HSAs offer another example. The two bodies' approaches to hospitals often talk entirely past one another; the HSA's findings about the community's "need" for hospital beds and facilities of one type or another have little concrete bearing on such quite distinct questions as whether the charges of hospital A are reasonably related to its costs of doing business, and whether or not that hospital is efficiently run. Moreover, HSA decision processes may seem to be offensively "soft" and "political" to the hard-nosed economists who staff or run many rate-setting bodies. The clearest case in point is Maryland, where officials of the state Health Services Cost Review Commission have publicly and often blasted the HSAs in their state for refusing to be tough and "economical" in their planning recommendations. The problem appears to be reduced when rate-setters have some planning background and HSAs assign a prominent role to economists on their staffs. However, when HSAs with relatively little economic expertise confront rate-setting bodies dominated by self-confident economists, interagency relations are apt to be chilly.

Bureaucratic Turf

The HSA mission is much closer to that of CON officials than it is to that of PSROs or rate-setters. The need assessments integral to the HSA planning process are expected to provide analytical foundation for CON decisions, and CON offices are required by the planning law to take account of HSA recommendations. One might therefore expect to find rather close cooperation between the two agencies.

HSA-CON relations differ significantly from state to state. At risk of overgeneralizing, however, there appear to be two broad patterns of interaction. First, the state may largely stand aside from HSA deliberations on CONs and rubber stamp the HSAs' work. Second, the state may (in the almost identical words of observers in two different states) let the HSAs do all the hard review work while reserving the actual decision for itself. The former pattern appears to be common among states that came relatively late to CON.[26] Where HSAs preceded or grew up alongside the CON program, they may keep strong hands on the process. In states that adopted CON well before the passage of the planning law, however, the second pattern is evident. In these states well-developed and entrenched CON staffs may resent Johnnies-come-lately invading their turf, upsetting their procedures, and adding new and seemingly uninformed voices to their reviews. That the HSA position on a proposed CON may be the result of deference to an assertive subarea council, or of a temporary truce between a SAC and a facilities review committee, does not increase the CON staff's confidence in HSA planning. And the localism of the HSA reviews may aggravate their fears. HSAs generally learn that they accomplish more by negotiating with would-be CON applicants early and informally, at preapplication stages, than by intervening later and facing a choice between acquiescence and public battling after the application has been submitted. Therefore the HSA may preempt consultation between the applicant and CON staff, may make representations about the likelihood and terms of approval that contradict CON staff's preferences, and may be allied with the applicant at later (that is, state-level) stages of review. For these reasons, CON staff may be reluctant to share "real" decision-making power with the HSAs.

Moreover, even if the HSA establishes harmonious relations with the CON staff in the CON office, fragmentation of planning and regulatory activities in some states can leave important decision points unaffected. In Massachusetts, for example, "the state health plan is prepared by the Office of State Health Planning, CON reviews are performed by the Determination of Need Office, and CON decisions are made by The Public Health Council."[27] The more fragmented the CON authority at the state level, the more numerous are the institutions with which the HSA must attempt to coordinate, and the more frequent are the opportunities for clashes of bureaucratic turf.[28]

These observations suggest the counterintuitive hypothesis that long state experience with health care regulation is not necessarily a precursor or predictor of smooth adaptation to *federal* planning and regulatory programs. Quite the contrary, new federal bodies may find less hospitality and coordination in states with a relatively long history of regulation--and the bureaucracies this implies--than in latecomers. Although early regulatory efforts indicate a greater *willingness* to regulate, the practical problem of meshing entrenched state bureaucracies with recently devised federal planning and regulatory agencies is not dispelled by a general consistency of mission.

Financing and Grant Patterns

It would seem intuitively obvious that an organization charged with comprehensive planning for the needs and resources of its jurisdiction must have, if its plans are to carry weight, some control, or at any rate leverage, over decisions about those needs and resources. But the fragmentation and heterogeneity of health insurance financing and grant-in-aid patterns in the United States place major elements of the needs-resources relationship beyond the HSAs' influence, let alone control. HSAs may express their opinions about the optimal numbers and distribution of physicians by specialty and place within their regions, but they can do little to influence the location and specialization decisions of physicians or the flow of federal manpower grants and loans to medical schools and students. They can do little to affect the big decisions about health benefits and premiums, which take place mainly in collective bargaining in the private sector. Medicare and Medicaid are entitlement programs, the one guaranteeing federal aid to the elderly, the other to the poor, for a range of medical services set forth in law. Furthermore, as one HSA put it, "the present method of reimbursement" in these programs "overshadows most local efforts at cost containment."[29] Resentful over alleged HSA discrimination against them, health maintenance organizations have fought free of much of the CON process.[30] Finally, as noted above, such federal regulatory efforts as PSROs and state efforts like rate-setting are usually far removed institutionally from health planning. In sum, in the words of Katharine

G. Bauer: ". . . the Planning Act excludes from the purview of the agencies it creates most of the key elements that currently determine the way the U.S. health system actually operates."[31]

The general point is a familiar one to organizational analysts: that two or more agencies labor in related fields and might in theory reap advantages from close cooperation does not automatically produce coordination.[32] A number of intervening organizational variables--one agency's ability to supply a product in demand by another, the agencies' definitions of their roles and missions, the sense of bureaucratic turf and priority, and administrative arrangements dividing fund flows between the public and private sectors and among levels of government--should be given careful consideration. For these and other reasons, interorganizational relations between HSAs and other health regulatory agencies will probably remain spotty for some time to come.

HSAs AND THE FEDERAL GOVERNMENT

For better or worse, the HSAs have not been left alone to founder in their intra- and interorganizational difficulties. HSAs are, after all, federal creatures, and the federal government, notably the Health Resources Administration (HRA) in the Department of Health and Human Services, has an organizational interest of its own in their success. As planning officials in the 10 federal regions contemplate their charges' progress to date, problems are evident and frustrations numerous. Some officials interviewed for this study were harshly frank. To summarize a frequently encountered critique: HSAs were created in 1974, often had the benefit of building on CHP foundations, receive hundreds of thousands (or more) of federal dollars annually, have sizable staffs-- and have done little more than assemble some warmed-over, highly general, and banal "plans" of little practical use to anyone. If the program is to shape up into a success, the regions need specific success stories to hold before HRA eyes in the central office, before secretarial eyes in HHS, and before congressional, General Accounting Office (GAO), Office of Management and Budget (OMB), and White House eyes. But how are such successes to be produced? Federal officials can exert little direct influence on "outcomes"; the only promising point of leverage is the plan itself. As the program has developed, central office regulations and guidelines, and therefore regional office instructions and pressures, have attempted to discipline the planning process, to require and coax the locals to make the plans more specific, rigorous, and quantitative, and then, in their CON and PUFF decisions, to follow the logic of the plan wherever it may lead. In this way, it is hoped, the planning process can be made to show "a demonstrable difference."[33]

In HSA eyes, however, federal rules and guidelines are at once offensively specific and unhelpfully vague. The locals suspect--correctly--that the feds have no better ideas about how to write health plans than they themselves do, and they therefore resent federal efforts to force an artificial consensus. Nevertheless, under the hot breath of the quantifying overseers, the feds have no choice but to insist, and the locals, eager to get their plans (and next year's grant award) approved with minimum conflict have no choice but to try--or to seem--to comply.

As one might expect, these downward pressures set off a complex chain reaction within the organizational structures of the HSA. Told by the feds to go back to the drawing board and improve their section of the plan, committees tend to grumble that a supposedly local planning process is being emasculated by domineering bureaucrats. At the same time the pressure tends to strengthen the hands of the staff, the repositories of methodological sophistication, and therefore of specificity, quantification, and rigor, and quite often the only ones who appear to understand the mumbo-jumbo the agency has been told to master. But when providers on the committees, SACs, or board then "test" the staff's proposed methodologies and quantified planning criteria against their own situations and institutional interests, they quickly identify distasteful results (for instance, a ward to be closed or not to be renovated after all) and with much noise and animation expose all the absurdities and anomalies of the mindless application of a general method or formula to an obviously exceptional case like their own. Letters from locals (angry) and feds (polite, reassuring, but firm) go back and forth. A federal regional planning expert or team is dispatched to meet with staff, executive director, and (perhaps) a few interested board members in order to help them understand "how to do it." The HSAs are given to understand that the content of their plans is, at least within broad limits, theirs to define as

they see fit. But whatever they do, they must do it
rigorously and specifically; the plan must be studded
with numbers, formulae, criteria, standards, and perhaps
even a few equations. HSA staff and committee members
then meet to thrash out a compromise that will be more
specific than what was contemplated before but still
hedged and ambiguous enough to be tolerable. The feds
withdraw, knowing that they have bought all the rigor the
local political market can produce. Plans that seem
better than the norm are called to HRA attention; the
agencies that wrote them attract "close interest." Top HHS
officials reassure OMB and the Congress that the planning
process is coming along, that many costs (including the
time and effort of local notables) have been sunk, and
that after all there really is no alternative to local
grass roots democracy when one wants cost containment
but abhors bureaucracy and government regulation. Even
as they receive their appropriations, however, these
officials worry that the budget-minded skeptics will
prevail next time, are acutely aware of the importance
of large, tangible (that is, quantifiable) results,
especially savings, soon, and increase pressure on the
regions to find such evidence. Regional pressures for
specificity, rigor, and measurement are in turn stepped
up, and HSAs again respond by putting staff, committees,
and SACs on the trail of compromises that quantify for
the sake of quantification, that is, for the sake of feds.

THE MYTHICAL FOUNDATIONS OF HEALTH PLANNING:
A CRITIQUE

The central problem with the HSA effort is that it rests
on theoretical foundations that cannot properly be
institutionalized--that is, embodied in structures that
effectively relate the planning strategy to the goals
it is intended to achieve. Three theoretical assumptions
are especially problematic.

Consumer-Dominated Pluralism

Cain and Darling write that:[34]

   One of the fundamental assumptions on which this . . .
   program is based is that a community of interest,

a set of shared perspectives, can be developed
between consumers and providers, insurance carri-
ers and policy holders, employers and employees,
town and gown, in the health sector. Out of
these shared perspectives, it is assumed Health
Systems Plans--and regulatory decisions--can
emerge. . . . To develop such shared perspectives,
all interests are to be represented on the planning agency boards--a majority of consumers, to
be sure, but an effective minority of providers
as well. . . .

The HSAs are to provide a forum in which diverse
social interests--divergent enough to be distinct and
even conflictual but not so divergent as to be beyond
reason and reconciliation--may come together and reach
compromises in the general public interest. "Provider
dominance," ever-feared and ever-impending, is to be
checked by provisions for a board with a majority of
consumers. Unfortunately, balance cannot be so easily
mandated. Consumer-dominated pluralism puts an excessive
burden on consumers, demanding that they walk a tight-
rope, neither deferring to providers nor becoming so
adversarial as to cease to be constructive. Somewhere
between capitulation and intractability lies the proper
consumer role. Alas, no one knows what this mythical
terrain looks like.
Although there is accumulating evidence on what
those occupying consumer roles do, there is very little
on how consumers tend to perceive and evaluate the health
care system.[35] It is therefore far from clear that many
consumers believe in, and are able to define and articulate, a consumer interest in health care clearly and
distinctly different from the interests of providers.
That consumers will ever take the lead in saying "no"
to expansion-minded providers in the name of regulatory
efficiency and cost-containment is highly doubtful.
Consumer participants, like other Americans, want to be
"constructive," not "negative," and they soon find that
the identification and elaboration of unmet needs and
the laying of plans to meet them is far more gratifying
than assaulting or undoing the plans of valued community
health resources such as hospitals. As Basil Mott put it,
"the HSAs, like the CHP agencies, will probably have
their greatest programmatic effect in encouraging and
assisting the development of desirable new programs. It

is easier to identify and agree on unmet needs and to
assist needed program development, especially when resources are available, than to change or discontinue already existing programs."[36] In the words of a consumer
coalition: "Most consumers enter health planning with
an eye turned toward specific issues: access, quality,
or more humane institutional alternatives."[37]

Consumer energies find four main outlets. First,
prevention, wellness, health education, health promotion,
holistic medicine, and the need to "encourage" these and
other fashionable movements stand high among the priorities
of many consumers. Providers may privately snicker at
these enthusiasms but they know that by joining in these
"promotions" they can win good will and allies in the
fights that count.

Second, consumers often emphasize relatively neglected
and "low technology" services--mental health counseling,
hypertension and diabetes management, pre- and post-
maternity care for mothers and children, and the like.
That improving these services may raise health care budgets, at least in the short run, is thought secondary.

Third, consumers may assail or try to block various
evils that local institutions have perpetrated. For
example, the Consumer Coalition quoted above boasts of an
HSA that "unearthed mammoth abuses and scandalous profit-
making by a dialysis company," of another that "discovered that a local hospital was building massage parlors
for its doctors and charging it off to consumers, third-
party payors, and Medicaid and Medicare," and of another
that investigated pharmacy pricing and uncovered kickbacks
to local doctors.[38] Hospitals that fail to meet their
obligations to Medicaid recipients or to provide enough
"free care" are another favored target. Institutions with
expansion plans that entail demolition of or eviction from
homes in adjacent neighborhoods are still another. In
these cases consumers may become skilled at using the regulatory leverage of the HSA--especially the certificate-
of-need review process--to bargain for institutional
"reforms."

It is difficult to evaluate these "reforms" because
they have not been studied closely and dispassionately.
They may arise from indefensible pressure applied by
uninformed and power-hungry citizens to administrators
trying to do a good job in trying circumstances. They
may bring about overdue correction of institutional indifference and neglect and may enhance the altruism and

moral fiber of local providers. Be this as it may,
they have little to do with cost containment.

Finally, consumers show some interest in cost containment. Sometimes this interest reflects their determination to punish a recalcitrant institution. Sometimes
it reflects a generalized hostility toward "high
technology" medicine. Sometimes it reflects staff influence, and sometimes a sincere commitment to a more
efficient and cost effective health care system. Approaches to "costing" based on a thoroughgoing assessment of resources in light of needs are seldom to be
found, however. For one thing, the issues involved--
which, to recall the consumer statement quoted earlier,
require "a merry chase through HSPs, AIPs, square footage
formulae, and debt ratios, etc."--are boring, dry, and
time-consuming. For another, consumers no more than
providers wish to see their area "lose ground" in the
competition for good health care resources. Consumers are
not, of course, indifferent to waste and inefficiency and
most have grasped that bedrock of American health planning,
Roemer's law. But Roemer's law, which holds, in essence,
that a bed built is a bed filled and which therefore
seems to point to constraints on or reductions in bed
capacity as a main route to cost containment, states a
general relationship, whereas HSA decisions are exercises
in the analysis of highly particular--indeed seemingly
unique--circumstances.[39] Direction is even more lacking
in decision-making about technology, for which, as Louise
Russell has remarked, there is no Roemer's law.[40] Health
planning confronts an unending parade of priorities; health
regulation faces an equally populous parade of exceptional
cases. This combination of unlimited need-listing and
indulgent exception-making does not conform to the clash
of distinctive interests pictured by the "countervailing
power" model of HSAs.

Even when consumers are inclined to get tough with
providers, the organizational setting in which they
must press their case is rarely conducive to persistence.
In the HSA committees and subarea councils, providers
worried about their own institutions, precedents, or "logs"
soon to be rolled are much more likely to attend meetings
and to participate knowledgeably and fully than are consumers. Four or five providers "versus" one or two
consumers are apt to prove highly persuasive. Those
who would employ small groups for planning purposes must
abide with the consequences of small group dynamics.

One of these consequences is a tendency for the groups to honor intensity of preferences, to sympathize with those members whose interests are clearly on the line and whose emotions are deeply engaged. These members are often the providers whose institutional excellence or character may be threatened. Another consequence is for community residents who expect to live, socialize, and work together over time to avoid and reduce conflict by means of deference and reciprocity.

It has been pointed out with justifiable celebration in some quarters, that despite the pessimism of early critics, the HSAs are "saying no" oftener than expected, that they are "doing more regulation" than predicted, and that consumers have frequently "bought" the need for cost containment with surprising dedication. All of this, it is said, represents the triumph of heroic public spiritedness over the true expansionist interests of local residents. There is no intention here to minimize this public-mindedness. The point of the argument developed here is rather that HSAs are a faulty cost containment mechanism *precisely because* they demand local public spiritedness in so high a degree.

Vast organizational anguish tends to accompany a "no" decision by an HSA on a question of genuine interest to a local health care institution. The many hours of negotiation; the recurrent cycle of justification and critique; the charges of lay ignorance on one side and of provider dominance on another; the endless fiddling with formulas and ratios no one understands; the contrived public hearings at which a hospital displays its audiovisual aids to testify to the urgent needs of a venerated community institution and "the community" in attendance (three-fourths of it employed by or related to employees of the hospital) rises in long-winded support; the 4-3 vote finally taken at 1 a.m. in committee; the endless buttonholing and hand holding; the threat of appeal and legal redress; all of this, inherent in self-regulating localism, raises the personal and organizational costs of nay-saying very high. Few care to go through this process very often. One may give the HSAs (especially their consumers and staffs) the credit they richly deserve for their firmness and still conclude that a local, highly participatory body is not the best means of making cost containing decisions, that nay-saying would be more reliably institutionalized at higher levels of the federal system.

Finally, consumers determined to fight for such cost
containing measures as denied expansion or modernization
projects, or for mergers or closures, may find that
their success in persuading the HSA board carries little
weight in the larger community. Tough HSA recommendations often come under sharp fire at public meetings
from contingents of "average citizens," some speaking
out spontaneously, others orchestrated by providers,[41]
and HSAs often back down under such fire. In short,
cost-conscious *consumer representatives* may find themselves at odds with the sentiments of *community participants*--a predicament to which enthusiasts of "greater
consumer representation and participation" have given too
little thought.[42]

It is unreasonable to mark out an independent and
separate consumer role and then expect consumers to conform to it because such a role is, at bottom, contrived
and unauthentic. Abstract and systemic health consumers
are nowhere to be found. People consume health care in
a great variety of very definite social contexts with
logics of their own--for example, as head of a family
worried about the health of a loved one; as resident of
a local community concerned about the distance to and
quality of hospital care should need arise; as a taxpayer
and wage earner considering the size of the annual federal
budget deficit, the effects of inflation, or the size of
a payroll deduction or of a wage increase foregone; as a
more or less informed layman contemplating the implications of some new technology--or the implications of Ivan
Illich; as personalities with certain attitudes toward
risk, pain, and one's own body; as members of local
organizations--unions, churches, hospital boards, and
auxiliaries, and so on--involved with health care institutions. There is no pure consumer role; even the most
resolutely skeptical citizen is compromised by emotions
and identifications that inhibit policital self-definition
as a "countervailing power" to "providers." (There are,
of course, "professional consumers" in the "Naderite"
sense. But in practice the role usually entails a deeper
and more consistent antagonism to providers than most
consumers are willing to adopt.)[43] The HSA effort partakes
of a central fallacy in current health policy analysis,
the determination to "decontextualize" the consumer, to
reduce him to pure *payer*, and then to expect him to
define and articulate a set of interests distinct from
those of the paid, the providers. Not surprisingly,

consumers continually violate these expectations, leaving their advocates fuming about provider dominance.

The unhappy fact is that there is no more agreement about the nature and purposes of the consumer role in health planning than there is about the nature and purposes of health planning itself. At least six distinct roles envisioned for consumer representatives may be culled from the literature and from legislative documents and debates. First, the representative role may be to express the community's viewpoint. A second role is to express the views of un- or underrepresented minorities or disadvantaged elements within the community. A third is to oppose--that is, "countervail"--the provider perspective. A fourth is to supplement--or perhaps supplant-- the positions of political officials. A fifth is to represent the stands of organizational constituencies. A sixth is to speak for those with special health care needs.

The various roles imply different recruitment procedures. The first, for example, would seem to call for a general election; the second and sixth, for quotas of different community strata; the third and fourth, for deliberate recruitment of those with distinct policy views (antiprovider and antipolitician, respectively); the fifth, for selection from among members or officers of formal organizations. And even if agreement about the proper meaning and method of recruitment of consumer representatives could be secured, an equally difficult problem--the relationship between consumer representation and community participation--would remain to be resolved. What is the legitimacy of recommendations made or decisions taken by consumer representatives on the HSA board but strongly opposed by consumer participants in the community itself?

It is idle to believe that the "proper" composition of HSA boards can be deduced from ever more sophisticated and refined philosophical, legal, and linguistic explications of the concept "consumer." The concept yields no such treasures. If the question at hand is whether (for example) working-class persons, or working-class Latinos, or working-class Latinos in need of kidney dialysis should be represented on the HSA board, then this question should be debated on its moral and political merits, not mired in linguistic analysis.

"Socially descriptive" representation is a particularly weak solution to the representative puzzle. In local health decision-making, representatives should represent their constituencies' *attitudes* (preferences) not merely their *attributes*. And one cannot directly infer attitudes from attributes. Many cleavages cut across such strata as class, race, neighborhood, ethnicity, health status, and so forth. Just as it was demeaning when the federal government incorporated in Great Society programs participation provisions based on the view that "the poor" and "the black community" are homogeneous, so too it is demeaning to assume that on health issues Latinos (or whomever) must be homogeneous in interest and attitude and may therefore be adequately represented by a (physical) Latino.

The familiar alternative--selecting consumer representatives from among the members or officers of consumer organizations--is no more clearly preferable, however. As Checkoway notes, consumer activism and organization in the health field do not conform to the traditional image of political mobilization boiling up from grievances deeply and widely felt in the community. Rather, the planning program itself and its institutional resources "have helped create career opportunities and support networks among activists and professionals seeking to identify issues and build organizations in a field in which consumers typically lack awareness of inequalities in the delivery of services, or do not accept health planning as a community problem, or show little support for consumer intervention."[44] This suggests the need for skepticism about whom and what self-proclaimed consumer groups represent. It is understandable that such groups argue that "To become responsible and responsive representatives, consumers need the technical and political support of an organized consumer health constituency,"[45] because wide acceptance of this view serves their organizational maintenance needs. There is a natural tension between socially descriptive representatives--especially elected and other prominent "group" figures--and organizational representatives over the "right" to speak for the consumer. Neither side is right; the representative limitations of both sides should be recognized.

Finally, notwithstanding the program designers' dim views of state and local politicians, one should ask what representative roles *these* figures properly play in health planning. Obviously, participation is in *some* sense a good thing in, indeed a defining feature of, a democracy, but a democracy is a hierarchy or polyarchy of diverse representative structures. Therefore, the general case for representation and participation implies nothing at all about the specific case for one or another approach to representation in health care policy. This point is usually ignored in discussions about consumer representation, which seem to assume that because participation is good one cannot have too much of it and that no proposal that appears to increase it can legitimately be faulted. Yet the issue remains: the community has "representatives"--elected officials-- and it may be unwise to forget them or usurp their roles or complicate their lives without first giving careful attention to the character of the polyarchy one creates by devising such supplementary--or supplanting--structures as the HSAs.

Because there is so little agreement about the content of the representative role, it is doubtful that any of these questions can be answered sensibly in the detailed language of statute, regulation, or court decision. Therefore, the present drift toward ever more detailed statutory, administrative, and judicial embroidery on the "true meaning" of consumer representation is unfortunate. The long and often unhappy history of similar efforts in urban policy--where requirements were diluted from "maximum feasible participation" in the community action program, to "widespread citizen participation" in the Model Cities program, to an "adequate opportunity to participate" in the Community Development Block Grant program[46] could teach health planners the futility of the search for uniform, correct, and precise definitions in this area, and may strengthen the case for increasing the discretion of the states and of the HSAs themselves in designing their consumer representation structures.

European practice offers some instructive contrasts. In continental Europe, consumers are represented neither by socially descriptive figures nor by self-constituted consumer organizations, but rather by organizations, the sickness funds, whose business it is to *purchase* health care. In West Germany, for example, most of the population is enrolled in occupation-related sickness funds. There are more than 1,000 separate funds, which compete to some extent--that is, within the constraints of legally required benefit packages--for members, especially for better-off and low-risk members. To retain their members, their reputations, and the better risks, the funds must offer an attractive package (extra benefits, perceived

quality, atmosphere, and so on) at rates that do not out-
rage the subscriber. (In West Germany half the cost of
coverage is paid by the employee and half by the employer.)
The funds must, therefore, bargain with physician organizations and with hospitals over fees and rates and have
developed large, expert staffs that match those of the
provider organizations in analytic and technical skill.[47]
The skills, numbers, and continuity of the sickness fund
bureaucracies supply the specialized leverage consumer
representatives in the United States generally lack.
Moreover, in Germany the workers sickness funds, which
enroll almost half the population, have close historical
ties to the labor unions and the (now ruling) Social
Democratic Party. These groups are a potentially powerful
legislative coalition that did, in fact, come together
successfully in 1977 to pass a cost containment law.[48]
Even so, the adequacy of consumer representation lies
very much in the eye of the beholder, and one recent
account describes its condition in the German health care
system as "bleak."[49]

It is doubtful that one can do much better, however,
and it is clear that the United States cannot now go
even this far toward institutionalized consumer representation. In the United States the sickness funds (Blue
Cross and commercial insurance companies) often represent
providers or shareholders more than consumers, a consequence of the circumstances of the birth and maintenance
of these organizations.[50] In the United States historical
ties among "progressive" parties, unions, and insurers
are largely absent too. It is, therefore, not surprising
that the United States tries to achieve consumer representation by mandating and designating consumer representatives on planning boards. But it is also not
surprising that this approach encounters many obstacles.

Some believe that European negotiating structures
contain a clear lesson for the United States: instead
of trying to spin from whole cloth new consumer representation bodies, policymakers should bring purchasers of
care more directly into decisions about health care rates
and charges. There are several problems with this
recommendation, of which two will be briefly noted here.
First, the fragmentation of the insurance industry in
the United States complicates representation in bargaining.
It is difficult to imagine how Blue Cross, Blue Shield,
private companies, HMOs, union plans, Medicare, Medicaid,
and still others could come together in the equivalent

of an "association of sickness funds" with leadership
speaking authoritatively for all members. Second, the
decentralization of health care regulation in the United
States further complicates the issue. Presumably much
of the bargaining would occur at the state level, where
the review and setting of hospital rates and the regulation of health insurance take place. It will do the
insurers little good to strike a bargain with providers
if there is no assurance that state regulators (rate-
setters, CON reviewers, and others) will abide by it.
Moreover, if "minority" insurance interests in a state
suspect that their larger and more powerful brethren
have cut a deal with state regulators at their expense,
bargaining may break down. In short, European negotiating
structures presuppose a national health insurance program
and a national health insurance statute that imposes
some unifying structure on the organization of the negotiating parties, on the nature of the bargaining process,
and on the allowable limits of subnational diversity.

Although the structural and organizational precondi-
tions of a disciplined, integrated pluralism in the
health field are not met here, the United States must
nonetheless try to make pluralism work. The American
medical and political systems are extremely fragmented.
Many interests are inescapably involved in health care
policy and some means must be found to bring them together on common ground. In Europe, where health care
financing takes place subject to public law and sometimes
with public funds, it is much easier for governments to
convene negotiations and to keep participants at the table.
The elements of the system come together in "health insurance bargaining"[51] between sickness funds and
providers, with unions, employers, government, and other
interested and highly organized parties standing on the
sidelines watching and prepared to influence and perhaps
even countermand the agreements of the two principal
negotiators. The U.S. health care system, by contrast,
is largely private, and even in its public sector it has
chosen to purchase care by cost- and charge-based retrospective reimbursement methods, not by means of rates
set forth prospectively in fee schedules. With arrangements so heterogeneous and decentralized, the United
States must experiment with heterogeneous and decentralized
frameworks for negotiation. The HSAs take halting steps
in this direction by establishing forums that bring
major interests into negotiations--over the contents of
the health plan.

Bargaining, however, is not a panacea. Creating forums in which providers and payers/consumers come together to negotiate is only half the job. The other half is the establishment of governmental rules and procedures that constrain bargaining, that is, set financial or other limits within which agreement must remain. The art of designing a workable negotiation system lies in finding the right balance between constraining structures imposed by government and bargaining autonomy enjoyed by providers and payers. This balance shifts with time and circumstance and must be intermittently modified.

In Europe, negotiations center not on the design of a comprehensive plan to address all facets of the health care system, but rather on a tangible and immediate financial question, the reimbursement levels for acts contained in the fee schedule. This in turn implies deliberation on the sources and definition of increases in the cost of medical and hospital practice, on the amount by which mandated contributions can be raised for employers and employees, and more. The structure of and participants in the bargaining process are prescribed in some detail by law, and government usually retains options such as extending existing fee levels indefinitely or (as in Germany) subjecting the two sides to compulsory arbitration, should negotiations break down.

In recent years health care cost increases have been very high and European governments have modified the structure of negotiations in ways that give them greater leverage. A West German law enacted in 1972, for example, gives the central government a larger role in the planning and financing of hospitals, a field in which the German states have jealously guarded their "rights." A 1976 law creates new planning mechanisms to influence the distribution of primary care. The cost containment law of 1977 created, among other central constraints, a multimember "concerted action" group at the federal level that makes annual recommendations on spending increases. Provider and sickness fund negotiators are expected (though not required) to keep their agreements within this ceiling. Stronger central "constraining structures" are widely seen to be necessary, though perhaps not sufficient, for cost containment.[52]

On occasion, European nations resort to localistic, roundtable planning methods. For instance, the West German law of 1976, addressing physician distribution, has several points of resemblance to the HSA process.[53]

It differs, however, in at least two major respects.
First, it aims not at comprehensive planning for the
system as a whole but rather at the analysis and cure
of a specific problem, physician distribution. Second,
it carries the threat of specific sanctions, if voluntary methods fail. (The law allows a committee of sickness funds and physician representatives, as a last
resort, to make establishment of new primary care
practices in overdoctored areas contingent on a permit.)
No European nation pretends that cost containment can
be achieved by means of localistic, vaguely defined
participatory processes and neither should the United
States.[54]

In Europe as in the United States, the complaint is
widespread that "providers dominate" the negotiating and
regulatory processes. However, it is doubtful that any
scheme can be devised in which full-time provider-experts
will not somehow dominate part-time consumer-laymen when
the two come together to plan for professional concerns.
This outcome is a function of widely shared values as
much as, probably more than, imbalances of power. The
choice lies not between provider and consumer dominance,
but rather between various structures and degrees of
provider-dominated systems. The reformer's task is to
discriminate carefully among these various structures
and inquire empirically into their consequences.

Self-Regulating Localism

The health planning effort assumes that assemblies of
local "interests" will regulate their health care demands,
acquisitions, and spending if only government gives them
a mandate and subjects them to the organizational structures of consumer-dominated pluralism. This assumption
is mistaken. Indeed one might argue that for planning
purposes the United States comprises two and only two
types of jurisdictions: those with adequate or excellent
health resources that they wish to preserve and enhance,
and those areas underserved in some respect, which hope
to gain more services and resources. The nostrum that
there is no constituency for cost containment is correct
only in part; it is by and large quite correct at the
local level, however.

The limitations of self-regulating localism are
especially evident in the case of hospitals, and not alone

in the United States. As William Glaser puts it in a
report on his research on European approaches to hospital
reimbursement:[55]

> One barrier against strict cost control over hos-
> pitals is the hesitation of the groups who other-
> wise are the watchdogs over health spending.
> The trade unions and sick funds resist higher
> fees for doctors but give hospitals the benefit
> of the doubt. The trade unions press for higher
> wages for hospital employees--the largest com-
> ponent of hospital costs--and oppose shutting
> small and underused hospitals. Sick funds try
> to relieve their own financial pressure by getting
> subsidies from government. Communities would
> rather have modern hospitals close at hand--even
> if underused--than save the tax money. Attempts
> by government to shut hospitals result in communi-
> ty protests and intervention by worried Parlia-
> ments, so that budget-cutters and planners often--
> not always--settle for a compromise. Hospital
> staffs are learning how to mobilize the community
> against ceilings on expenditures in particular
> services. . . .

One explanation of the lack of local taste for self-
regulation is that no local actor has any objective
interest in trying to limit or take away health resources
from his jurisdiction. As Harvey Sapolsky and others
have explained, the jurisdictions of those who benefit
from community health care resources and of those who
pay for them are rarely equivalent.[56] Nor are HSAs
obliged to plan within a ceiling, that is, a fixed health
budget, so that more of x must mean less or none of y.
    More research is needed into the perceptual roots of
local indifference to cost containment. Perhaps this
attitude does indeed reflect the calculated false
economizing of "free riders." But perhaps the roots are
more subtle. After all, everyone pays for health ser-
vices--in higher premiums, taxes, payroll deductions,
prices, and otherwise--and everyone knows it. But just
as an attitude of general support for national health
insurance or school integration may break down when the
supporter is questioned about concrete proposals (the
health security plan, or the prospect of busing, for
instance), so too a general commitment to cost containment

may collapse when planners get down to local cases.
Every student of budgeting understands this disjunction
between general principle and particular application:
of course less of the federal budget should be spent on
health care; but the proper place to make cuts is obviously not the Institutes of Health or Medicaid, or
the Cooperative Health Statistics System, or the health
planning program, and so on.

The response, in other words, depends heavily on
how the question is posed. The premise behind self-
regulating localism is that central government is the
appropriate level at which to pose general questions
(about the need for cost containment, for example), but
that the local level is the proper site of specific
decision-making. But the supposedly indispensable
insight, the unique wisdom, of local planners about local
needs and preferences usually argues for "more and
better" or at any rate for "no less and no worse." Thus,
a workable regulatory approach may require reversing
the usual premise: central and perhaps state government
may need to exploit the abstract and *general* agreement
at the local level on the need for cost containment
in order to force or constrain *specific* decisions that
localities would not voluntarily (that is, apart from
steady federal pressure or rules) reach by themselves.

It is often argued that visiting the true costs of
health services more accurately on those who reap the
benefits would lead to cost containment without additional governmental intervention. This could be done
in two ways. First, "individual" approaches seek to
make service recipients responsible for more of the health
care costs they incur. Second, "areal" efforts seek to
introduce a larger measure of jurisdictional equivalence
between communities of those who receive and of those
who pay for services.

European experience is again suggestive. The West
German system, for example, has a high degree of individual
targeting of costs: beneficiaries (that is, employees and
their dependents) pay half the cost of health care premiums through payroll deductions. In recent years average
contribution rates have climbed from about 8.5 percent
(1969) to more than 11 percent (1976) of income,[57] yet
despite some grumbling there has been no outpouring of
popular discontent and no major cuts in the very generous
benefits Germans enjoy.[58]

Sweden, by contrast, has a high degree of areal cost
targeting. Hospitals are supported mainly from county

budgets raised by county taxes. Indeed hospitals are
by far the largest single item in county tax levies,
which would presumably make their costs highly visible
and controversial. Yet Swedes have, on the whole, cheerfully raised county taxes to meet rising hospital costs.[59]

In Germany, Sweden, and elsewhere rapidly rising
health care costs have been "viewed with alarm," mainly
by the central government, not by public opinion or
localities, and central governments have been the major
source of cost containment efforts. This is not surprising: whereas an individual or a locality may evaluate
health care costs in a rough and intuitive judgment about
whether a payroll deduction or tax bill seems "fair
enough" in light of benefits conferred, central budget
makers must contemplate the extrapolation of present
health spending trends to truly horrifying percentages
of GNP and of social budgets within a decade or two and
must responsibly consider the opportunity costs of health
expenditures. The implications are that effective regulation is incompatible with extreme decentralization of the
regulatory body; that it is naive to expect that in the
United States more decentralization will cure problems
to which decentralization in large measure gives rise;
and that serious efforts at cost containment must come not
from self-regulating local bodies but from the central or
perhaps state government. Of course the central government
must and will involve localities in the design and implementation of cost containment plans, but this involvement
presupposes a strong, constraining, centrally established
framework. Programs like the HSAs, all involvement and no
(or very little) framework, can be expected to accomplish
few savings.

Scientifically Grounded Planning

The HSA effort is above all a health "planning" process
and the health plans stand at the center of the enterprise.
The plans are, so to speak, both output and input: *devising* plans that are both comprehensive and specific is
the first object of the exercise; *using* those plans to
guide regulatory decisions then follows.

Unfortunately, the substantive knowledge needed to
support plans of great comprehensiveness and specificity
in the health care field is lacking.[60] "The agency must
consider the array of influences on health," indeed it

must identify "all relevant health factors and problems."[61]
These "influences," "factors," and "problems" are easy
enough to list, but the practical component of the exer-
cise--"where possible isolate those conditions that can
be addressed by the delivery system"--is hotly disputed.
Equally important, the *relative* contributions of different influences, factors, and problems to health under
different conditions are poorly understood.

The same problems beset the instruction that the plan
should "describe and characterize the status of the entire health system. . . ."[62] If this means making a
list of institutions, services, and resources, it is a
feasible (though not easy) task. But the second part of
the mandate--"noting the effects that changes in one
part of the system may have on other parts"--can at best
be met with long lists of controverted propositions and
counterpropositions; meaning, hypotheses; meaning, con-
jectures. Third, and most important, the interactions between the two realms--the set of interacting factors that
produce or damage health and the set of interacting institutions that constitute the health care system--are
not well understood. It follows then, fourth, that many
other questions central to the HSA effort--for example,
the relative contributions of various factors and institutions to health care *costs,* and the degree to which costs
incurred do or do not "buy health"--cannot be answered
with more than educated guesses either.

The designers of the program were not content with
best guesses. They seem to have believed that the HSAs
could either consume the fruits of or generate scientific
research that would, once incorporated in the plans, provide a basis for scientific regulation. Decision-making
would consist of the application of demonstrated propositions to particular cases so as to yield an entirely
reasoned and nonarbitrary finding. But in most cases
either there exists no general proposition that has been
proved beyond dispute or the juxtaposition of general
proposition and particular facts fails to yield a single,
logical, determinate solution. The plan may be made
comprehensive by compiling exhaustive lists of factors,
institutions, and hypothesized relationships. It may be
made sophisticated by discussing the evidence for and
against major hypotheses. But it cannot also be simultaneously scientific and specific in its regulatory
applications. The expected smooth transition between
plan as product and plan as regulatory input is anything
but smooth.

Even if the intellectual demands of scientific planning were met, the institutional demands probably could not be. Planning of such scale and complexity must be broken down into special work units. This division of labor may, as illustrated above, lead to coordination problems among differently oriented elements within the planning organization itself. This problem, which can greatly hamper the work even of coordinating organizations with relatively clearcut and focused goals,[63] is of key importance to the HSAs. Their mission is too broad, complex, and unfocused for easy institutionalization and can be institutionalized only at the price of a continual struggle, often abandoned or lost, for an agencywide, "comprehensive" agenda.

It is a myth that regulation must or can be based on a wide range of scientific propositions integrated in plans. Regulation inevitably involves a large measure of educated guesswork--that is, holding the regulated to standards based on "best-available" or "suggestive," but not conclusive or airtight, evidence. That regulation is inevitably "arbitrary" to some extent does not mean, notwithstanding the language of the Administrative Procedures Act, that it is also necessarily "capricious." Steps to ensure that the guessers and the guesses are as educated as possible, that administrative procedures for exception-making and redress exist, and that the promulgators of the statutes, rules, or decisions containing the regulations have the obligation and opportunity to review them periodically in light of new evidence and in light of accumulating experience with their workings in the real world, offer safeguards.[64] So, too, do the negotiating forums working within these regulatory constraints. This, alas, is the best a government determined to contain health care costs can do. Science will no more generate a planned solution than the market will yield an unplanned one.

"REFORMS" IN THE PLANNING PROGRAM

What might be done to improve the HSA process? The arguments developed above suggest that the structural reforms now under discussion will make little difference. For example, some recommend a reduction in the role of the federal government, especially the federal bureaucracy, and would even turn the planning process over to the

states in the form of health revenue-sharing or block
grant funds. To be sure, federal efforts to mandate
rigor without offering practical advice on how to fulfill
this mandate have their costs. As noted above, the
emphasis on quantification and technique tends to bore
and intimidate consumers, confining debate increasingly
to staff, who seem to grasp the conceptual complexities,
and providers, who grasp the importance of making sure
that whatever the latest proposed formulas and criteria
may mean, they will not mean less for their institutions.
But these pressures also have their benefits. They
stem from the accurate belief that many HSAs, left on
their own, would write plans so general and vague that
virtually nothing--no acquisition or expansion request,
no proposed federal grant--would ever be "inconsistent"
with them. In regulation a start must be made somewhere:
standards and criteria that seem to be, on the whole,
reasonable must be negotiated, adopted, tried out,
and then retained, fine-tuned, or abandoned in the light
of experience. Federal officials and HSA planners may
speak of scientific rigor, but they settle in practice (as
they must) for applications of conventional wisdom and
common sense to local situations. Even this is accomplished only by considerable arm-twisting and consensus-
forcing, and it is questionable whether HSAs are the right
institutional locus for such consensus-forcing. But if
the nation is determined to retain HSAs with a regulatory
role, then some federal consensus-forcing should be
retained too.

Even if one cheerfully relieved the federal bureaucracy
of all participation in the program, all the major difficulties of the HSAs would remain. Federal pressures have
generally aimed to influence the *form* of local planning,
more than its substance; the lack of substance in many
HSA plans has little to do with the federal government.
The basic problems--making practical sense of an ambitious
mission, managing the subunits of a complex organization,
influencing related programs over which HSAs have no power,
devising a "proper" consumer role, generating a local
constituency for cost containment, drawing and applying
comprehensive plans in the absence of the substantive
knowledge such plans demand, and more--would all remain
severe in a devolved health planning program.

A second school of structural reformers would strengthen
the role of the HSAs vis-à-vis their organizational en-
vironment--the PSROs, CON staffs, rate-setters, SHPDAs,
and SHCCs. One can imagine any number of formal clearance

mechanisms obliging PSROs, CON staffs, and rate-setters
to take fuller account of HSAs: memoranda of understanding,
coordinating liaisons and councils, review and sign-off
requirements, and more come readily to mind. Forced to
confront the facts of bureaucratic life, however--dis-
crepancies in definitions of role, mission, and "distinctive competence"; struggles over bureaucratic turf; diverse
channels of financing and grants-in-aid; and the relatively low utility of many HSA plans to date--these formal
clearance mechanisms will probably generate paperwork
and little more.[65] It may be expected that the views and
works of the HSAs will be treated with respect by other
agencies when, and only when, they address these agencies'
concerns pertinently, and in their (the agencies') terms.
This happy day may never come, and federal interorganizational coordination-forcing is unlikely to hasten its
arrival.

Conversely, some would argue not for greater HSA
leverage over state-level decisions, but rather for greater
state influence on HSA decisions. If the basic problem
is that the HSA approach "places the primary responsibility
for planning at the substate regional levels" and thereby
"gives precedence to local perspectives . . ." whereas
"most if not all of the problems require statewide and
national perspectives to be seen in their true dimensions,"[66] then why not work to strengthen statewide
perspectives? A proper discussion of this question lies
beyond the scope of this essay. A quick illustration,
however, suggests that this is easier said than done.
Some indication of the potential and limits of strong
state leadership may be gained from recent events in
Michigan. In most states, the HSA process is highly fragmented. In Michigan, however, influence is more easily
concerted. There the major political actors--the "big
three" auto companies and the United Auto Workers (UAW)--
have expressed much public concern about cost containment
and joined with Blue Cross to persuade the legislature to
adopt a law calling for bed closures in the near future.
This approach has been described as the most stringent
assault on excess beds made to date in the United States.
It is doubtful that this "interest group centralization"
can be duplicated in many other states, however; the so-
ciopolitical structure of Michigan is in these respects
highly distinctive.

Adopting the plan and implementing it are two different
matters, moreover. The HSA covering Detroit appointed a
29-member commission to devise a bed reduction plan

in its jurisdiction. These efforts immediately evoked
charges of racism from black physicians, from hospital
officials, and from members of the black community, eager
to protect institutions on their own turf.[67] The
state then postponed implementation of the Detroit reduction while it considered the question anew. Early in
1980 a key participant gave his summary evaluation of
HSA planning in the atypically ambitious and rigorous
context of the Michigan law in these words: "These
days I use the time driving into Detroit for the HSA
meetings outlining the book I'm going to write about the
health planning process: I'll call it 'Anatomy of a
Failure.'"

An alternative to ambitious bed reduction legislation
is a strong determination of state officials to get
deeply involved in HSA planning and to hold the HSA's
feet to the fire. This too is easier said than done.
The same problems of regulatory equity now troubling
Detroit arise wherever a state government makes a serious
effort to close hospitals serving the poor, usually the
black poor, in central city areas. New York State has
been uncommonly aggressive in its efforts to close down
"unneeded" hospitals in New York City and it has usually
enjoyed the support of the city's mayor. "The community,"
however, has taken a different view and, aided by the
local HSA, by lawsuits, by eleventh hour federal money,
and in other ways, has fought to prevent these closings.

Moreover, state activism can lead, ironically, to
elaborate and possibly dysfunctional applications of the
"law of anticipated reactions." For example, some observers argue that the knowledge that the state will
have the final word on CON reviews encourages HSAs to
avoid starting fights with local providers. If an
unusually poor or unjustified project goes through, "the
state" will raise objections--and take the heat. Yet
HSA planners, who may happily defer to the state, then
complain vociferously that the state has emasculated and
mocked what was intended to be a local process when
these more central actors question their work.[68]

Third, one may envision a number of reforms in the
present organizational structure of health planning. If,
as argued here, the effort is too decentralized and
participatory to work well, one might consider some
structural variations that alter the organizational
character of the planning agency, the level of government at which planning occurs, or both. A highly

decentralized, weakly bureaucratized planning approach
is not the only option. For example, planning may be
decentralized but highly bureaucratized, as is much city
("master") planning. The problem here is that unless
the bureaucrat-planners and their product enjoy the
confidence of their political superiors, their plans will
gather dust on a shelf.[69] Planning may be highly centralized, but relatively nonbureaucratic, as was the
Office of War Mobilization and Reconversion, described
by Herman Somers.[70] This presidential agency made
decisions of great importance with a small, hard-working
staff headed by an executive (James Byrnes) who enjoyed
the highest presidential trust. But this was a wartime
expedient, terminated as soon as the war ended, and no
one proposes anything like it in the health care field
today. There are highly centralized and highly bureaucratic arrangements such as the wage and price control
bodies established in the Nixon administration.[71] The
problems encountered here--bureaucratic inflexibility or
seeming arbitrariness in the face of an endless parade
of requests for exceptions to general rules--are
essentially the opposite of those encountered in the HSAs--
an inability to formulate general rules and a cheerful
willingness to concede exceptions to such rules as are
devised.

These "alternatives" offer little more than mental
exercise, but this exercise recalls a simple but important
point: the decision to avoid larger measures of centralization and bureaucracy in health planning at once reflects
important social values and entails certain social costs.
The HSA approach offers the satisfaction of responsive-
ness--"doing something"--at the price of effectiveness,
that is, substantive accomplishment.[72] In health care as
in other fields, the confident term "planning" conceals
a multitude of hesitations and confusions.

Finally, a modest structural change worth considering
is to introduce a more rational division of labor in the
HSAs by changing the sequence of interaction of the participants and the roles they play. The current practice
essentially entrusts all tasks to all participants;
activities are divided up largely as the participants
choose, but in ways that preserve a roundtable mix of
consumer and provider interests at each stage. However,
one might consider matching tasks to the strengths of
the participants. For example, one might borrow a principle from the theory of legislative-executive relations:
the more expert branch (the executive, at the head of the

bureaucracy) should initiate proposals and do the detail-
work; the less specialized, more common-sensical, more directly accountable branch (the legislative) should review
("oversee") and amend these proposals from the layman's
viewpoint. Applying this principle to the planning process, one might argue that providers, who have expertise,
professional legitimacy, detailed institutional knowledge,
and intensity of preferences on their side, should initiate, that is, draw up first drafts of local health plans.
Then, consumers and representatives of special groups
might review the drafts, press questions, hear the appeals
of disaffected providers, and negotiate over additions,
deletions, and changes. It might be a good thing to endow
the consumer "side" with a sizable professional staff of
its own. (This, for example, was an early and insistent
demand of citizen participants in the Model Cities program. The neighborhood representatives were convinced,
probably correctly, that they could not hope to keep pace
with municipal "providers"--agencies--unless they had a
staff of their own.) State government could stand by as
an arbitrator, with authority to devise a plan of its
own if the locals failed to reach agreement within a
reasonable time. Both state and federal approval of
the plans would be required, giving these governments some
bargaining leverage too. This approach offers a more
reasonable division of labor than the present mingling
of skills at every stage. It arrives at decisions by
a structured sequence of planning, review, negotiation,
amendment, and approval, not by roundtable discussions that
leave the final word to large, part-time, and often unco-
hesive boards and SHCCs.

Structural changes might improve the planning process
at the margin, but no one should expect them to affect
fundamentally the problems from whith HSAs now suffer.
Their basic problems lie not in their structures but
rather in the breadth, heterogeneity, and complexity of
their mission. As long as the HSAs are asked simultaneously to be research, planning, regulatory, and advocacy
bodies, their way will not be smooth. As long as they are
asked to assume these four roles *and* to make a "demonstrable difference" in costs, in the delivery system, in
health status, in access (and so on and on), they will be
bound to disappoint.

Then why not change their missions? In particular, why
not distinguish the "academic" functions of research, planning, and perhaps advocacy from regulation and relieve the
HSAs of responsibility for the latter? Almost everyone

agrees that the HSAs "need time" to pull themselves
together and show results. But the regulatory component
of the mission robs them of time by insistently flinging
down the gauntlet of "demonstrable differences." HSAs
could instead be treated as "merit goods," as community
debating, deliberating, and consensus-building associations, as not-all-that-expensive luxuries that an indulgent society can easily afford.

Furthermore, it is doubtful that even endless grants
of time and money will turn the HSAs into effective
regulators. Regulation, it was argued above, demands not
consumer-dominated pluralism, but exertions of political
will; not self-regulating localism, but a strong measure
of detachment from the local milieu, that is, a greater
measure of centralization at the federal (and perhaps
at the state) level; not scientifically grounded planning,
but rather a determination to translate best-reasonable
guesses into laws and regulations and then remain
sensitive to the need for change. On each count, the
presuppositions of the HSAs place regulation on precisely
the wrong footing. If the HSAs need relief from regulation, regulation equally needs relief from the HSAs.

But something might be lost after all from such relief.
Although no sensible observer would contend that the HSAs
have much improved people's health, dramatically increased access to care, or (still less) saved the system
much money, they do appear to be making, at least in
some places, three less flamboyant contributions. First,
they have exerted themselves on behalf of neglected
areas and "priorities" of medical service--mental health,
prevention, ambulatory care, and so on--that find few
strong institutional advocates among local organizations.
Second, they have put pressure on local institutions,
especially hospitals, to devote more resources, attention,
and sympathy to the needs of the poor. And third, they
apply countervailing power against various elites contending
for dominance over health care policy.

This third point deserves brief amplification. *Governmental* elites at all three levels of government are mainly
concerned with saving money albeit without "too much"
regulation or other causes of aggravation. *Analytic*
elites, based mainly in the academic community, clamor
for the chance to apply in public policy their latest
syllogism purporting to demonstrate that (by means of
market approaches, competition, incentives, or whatever)
much money can be saved with no threat to access, to quality, or to other legitimate ends. *Provider* elites argue

for their professional autonomy and for high levels of remuneration. *Consumer* elites in proliferating consumer protection organizations claim a unique legitimacy in representing the voice of the average man and woman in health policy questions.

These elites respond to budgetary, intellectual, professional, and organizational incentives and maintenance needs, respectively. They are liable to be swept up in their particular perspectives and interests and lose touch with popular opinion. The HSA process reminds these elites that out there amidst the common folk there is still more interest in access than in efficiency, in preserving and equalizing than in cost cutting. This contribution has little to do with cost containment, but the HSAs' ability to make it probably depends importantly on preserving the limited regulatory leverage they now enjoy. Without a formal voice in grant reviews, their views on local medical priorities might not be heard. Without the power to delay and bargain over CON applications, they might be unable to pressure local hospitals into doing more for the poor. Without the presumption that the local plan stands for and is to be used for something, contending elites might find it convenient to ignore local sentiment.

There is of course irony in the observation that agencies endowed with regulatory powers in hopes that they would use them to strike a blow for cost containment are using them partly to contain the cost containers,[73] and there is double irony in the contention that they may need to retain regulatory powers precisely to enable them to go on striking blows that probably raise health care costs. Perhaps then the proper policy response is finally to throw irony over in favor of logic. After all, there are other, better, more equitable ways of honoring neglected priorities and groups than by means of local organizational pressure: by committing new federal money to support these priorities and by extending, refining, and enforcing the legal entitlements of Medicaid recipients, for example. And although there may be nothing like a grass roots organization to ex- press grass roots sentiment, this is not the last word in representation. A pluralistic, federal system like the United States has *layers* of representation and it is far from obvious which layer or mix of layers is most suitable to represent public opinion on a given policy question.[74] Who is to say that the localities' concern

45

with keeping their underused maternity wards alive
and well should be treated as a more authoritative,
representative datum than the concern of a U.S. president
or congressional committee with the frightening growth of
health care expenditures over time? One need not pose
policy questions so as to elicit highly detailed local
preferences, and sometimes one should not.

The unwieldy, delegated mission of the HSAs is vivid
testimony to failures of political will at the federal
level, failures that themselves reflect an absence of
consensus in society about the content of desirable
health care policies. It may therefore be a good idea
to retain the HSAs much as they are as a reminder, a
mirror, of this confusion and ambivalence. Perhaps some-
time in the future the nation will come to view health
care costs as a problem grave enough to justify the
adoption of "real" regulation. A final irony, then: the
HSAs may begin to "work" only after the federal government
wraps them in a regulatory framework that will render
them largely superfluous.

NOTES

The research on which this paper draws was supported by
grant number HS 02932 from the National Center for Health
Services Research, OASH. The author is grateful for the
valuable comments of Robert Derzon, William Glaser, Adela
J. Gondek, Charyl Kiger, Bonnie Lefkowitz, Louise Russell
and Jessica Townsend on an earlier draft, and to col-
leagues at the Institut für Medizinische Informatik
and Systemforschung (MEDIS) in Munich for explaining the
rudiments of the West German health care system during
the summer of 1980. Views advanced in this paper are the
author's and should not be attributed to these individuals
or to the officers, trustees, or other staff members of
The Brookings Institution.

1. As Christa Altenstetter points out: "During the
past 25 years or so, comparative studies on political
systems . . . have focused attention on politics and
processes, assuming that *structure* had little or no influence in shaping these processes. . . ." *Health
Policy-Making and Administration in West Germany and the
United States* (Beverly Hills: Sage Publications, 1974),
p. 8, italics in original.

2. The phrase is taken from Martha Derthick, *The Influence of Federal Grants* (Cambridge, Mass.: Harvard University Press, 1970).

3. The organization-building strategy has also been prominent in federal health efforts other than planning. Neighborhood health centers, health maintenance organizations, and professional standards review organizations are the leading additional examples.

4. U.S. Department of Health, Education, and Welfare, Health Resources Administration, "Directory: Health Systems Agencies, State Health Planning and Development Agencies, Statewide Health Coordinating Councils," November 1, 1979.

5. For elaboration, see George Gregory Raab, *Health Planning and American Federalism* (Ph.D. dissertation, University of Virginia, 1980).

6. As it turned out, the planning law and regulations granted very considerable powers to the states. See *ibid.* and Drew Altman, "The Politics of Health Care Regulation: The Case of the National Health Planning and Resources Development Act," *Journal of Health Politics, Policy, and Law,* vol. 2 (1978), pp. 560-580, especially pp. 565-572.

7. The phrase is taken from Charles Lindblom, *The Intelligence of Democracy* (New York: The Free Press, 1965).

8. "A pervasive belief underlying the legislation is that planning is a mechanistic enterprise, a matter of developing and applying technical expertise. The central process of mechanistic planning is the development of objective, numerical standards to rationalize the health facilities system and to determine scientifically the correct health care investments to be made." Randall Bovbjerg, "Problems and Prospects for Health Planning: The Importance of Incentives, Standards, and Procedures in Certificate of Need," *Utah Law Review,* vol. 3 (1978), pp. 83-121, quotation at p. 93.

9. Bruce C. Vladeck, "Interest-Group Representation and the HSAs: Health Planning and Political Theory," *American Journal of Public Health,* vol. 67 (1977), pp. 23-29; see also, Basil J. F. Mott, "The New Health Planning System," in Arthur Levin (ed.), "Health Services: The Local Perspective," *Proceedings of the Academy of Political Science,* vol. 32 (1977), pp. 238-254; and Aaron Wildavsky, "Can Health Be Planned?" 1976 Michael M. Davis Lecture, Center for Health Administrative Studies, Graduate School of Business, The University of Chicago.

10. Harry P. Cain II and Helen B. Darling, "Health

Planning in the United States: Where We Stand Today,"
Health Policy and Education, vol. 1 (1979), p. 10.
   11. *Ibid.,* pp. 15-16.
   12. The Codman Research Group, Inc., *Health Planning
and Regulation: The New England Experience, Final
Report,* vol. 1, part 1 (September 30, 1979), p. 70.
(Hereafter cited as "Codman Report.")
   13. Mott, "The New Health Planning System," p. 24.
   14. Barry Checkoway, "Consumerism in Health Planning
Agencies," January 1981, p. 160 (in this volume).
   15. A good example is the recurring argument over
the merits of process versus outcome measures in health
planning. See the discussion in Downs' paper in this
volume.
   16. Mott, "The New Health Planning System," p. 244.
   17. In recent amendments, however, "A consumer
majority is required for all subcommittees or advisory
bodies appointed by an HSA governing board or executive
committee." U.S. Department of Health, Education, and
Welfare, Health Resources Administration, "Health Planning Amendments of 1979: A Summary," n.d., p. 5.
   18. Many staff soon turn to practicing these skills
in the private sector. As the Codman Report (p. 40) ob-
serves: "The turnover is high on HSA staffs and in
state agencies with the forwarding addresses often being
state hospital associations, PSROs or major hospitals.
The first head of certificate of need review in Massachusetts left to join a Boston teaching hospital. Her
successor recently quit also, taking a post at a major
suburban community hospital. Their colleague responsible
for the preparation of planning standards is now with the
hospital association in an adjoining state. Several HSA
staff members also now work for hospital councils or local
providers. No one can say judgments of regulators are
compromised by the prospects of future employment with
the industry; no one can say they are not either."
   19. The list is taken from Lorabeth Lawson, "Evaluation of the Performance on HSA's in Region X and Implications for Future Technical Assistance Efforts: Summary
Findings," Discussion Paper no. 13, Center for Health
Services Research, Department of Health Services, University of Washington, April 1979, p. 4. (Hereafter cited
as "Performance of HSA's in Region X.")
   20. *Ibid.*
   21. Consumer Coalition for Health, "Written Submission to the Institute of Medicine Panel on Consumer Participation in Health Planning," April 9, 1980, pp. 4-5,
italics in original.

22. Health Planning Resources Development Amendments of 1974, H. Rept. 190, 96 Cong. 1 Secs. (GPO, 1979), p. 36.

23. Lawson, "Performance of HSA's in Region X," pp. 11-13, quotation at p. 11.

24. *Ibid.*, p. 14.

25. The terms "definition of role and mission" and "distinctive competence" come from Selznick's *Leadership in Administration* (New York: Harper and Row, 1957), p. 42 and ch. 3.

26. When the health planning law was enacted in 1974 about half the states had certificate-of-need laws.

27. Codman Report, p. 76.

28. On problems of coordination arising from multiple clearance points, see Jeffrey Pressman and Aaron Wildavsky, *Implementation* (Berkeley: University of California Press, 1973), especially ch. 5.

29. "Statement of the Florida Gulf Health System Agency on Consumer Participation in Health Planning," presented to the Committee on Health Planning Goals and Standards of the Institute of Medicine, National Academy of Sciences, Washington, D.C., March 27, 1980, p. 3.

30. P.L. 96-79, section 1527.

31. Katharine G. Bauer, *Cost Containment Under PL 93-641: Strengthening the Partnership Between Health Planning and Regulation,* Harvard University Center for Community Health and Medical Care, Report Series R58-8, January 1978, p. 29.

32. See *ibid.* for an extensive discussion of these problems in the programs discussed here.

33. Cain and Darling, "Health Planning in the United States," p. 23.

34. *Ibid.*, p. 21.

35. In general, public opinion polls offer the rather unhelpful findings that the citizenry is quite satisfied with the U.S. health care system but nonetheless worried about its costs, access, manpower, and the like; that many citizens favor national health insurance in general, but not any one proposal in particular; and so forth. The polls furnish no basis at all for judging how public opinion would address the central practical policy problem, making trade-offs among "goods."

36. Mott, "The New Health Planning System," p. 251. See, however, the Codman Report, pp. 54-61, or Altman, "The Policy of Health Care Regulation," pp. 573-576, for the view that the HSAs are doing "more regulation than expected."

37. Consumer Coalition for Health, "Written Submission . . . ," p. 5.

38. *Ibid.*

39. On the difficulties in the way of rigorous application of "need" and other criteria to certificate-of-need reviews, see Harold S. Luft and Gary A. Frisvold, "Decisionmaking in Regional Planning Agencies," *Journal of Health Politics, Policy, and Law,* vol. 4 (1979), pp. 250-272.

40. Louise B. Russell, *Technology in Hospitals* (Washington: The Brookings Institution, 1979), p. 140.

41. Codman Report, pp. 61-67.

42. See Bruce C. Vladeck, "Health Planning--Participation and Its Discontents," *American Journal of Public Health,* vol. 69 (1979), pp. 331-332.

43. Consumer representatives may empathize with a health care consultant who recounted his "worst nightmare": he is addressing a body of local physicians, flailing the waste and inefficiency of fee-for-service medicine, only to be stricken in mid-sentence with a heart attack and then saved by members of his audience.

44. Checkoway, "Consumer Movements in Health Planning," p. 180.

45. *Ibid.,* p. 178.

46. On the OEO experience see Daniel P. Moynihan, *Maximum Feasible Misunderstanding* (New York: The Free Press, 1970). On Model Cities see Lawrence D. Brown and Bernard J. Frieden, "Rulemaking by Improvisation: Guidelines and Goals in the Model Cities Program," *Policy Sciences,* vol. 7 (1976), pp. 455-488, especially pp. 464-474. The language quoted from the Housing and Community Development Act of 1974 appears in P.L. 93-383, Section 104.

There are many striking similarities between the Model Cities program and the planning effort: the emphasis on planning and coordination, the determination to pursue them by means of a newly built local organization, the deep concern with citizen participation, the federal attempt to make the planners follow a rigorous sequence of goal-setting, problem analysis (and so on) resulting in long-term and short-term plans, the problems of reconciling the powers of the new organization with those of local public officials and with the interests of local organizations, both public and private, and more. Unfortunately, academics and public officials have apparently made little effort to learn from the difficulties of

the Model Cities program lessons of practical advantage
to the HSAs. On Model Cities see Lawrence D. Brown,
*Coordination of Federal Urban Policy: Organizational
Politics in Three Model Cities* (Ph.D. dissertation,
Harvard University, 1973).

47. On Europe, see William A. Glaser, *Health Insurance Bargaining: Foreign Lessons for Americans* (New
York: Gardner Press, 1978); Howard M. Leichter, *A
Comparative Approach to Policy Analysis: Health Care
Policy in Four Nations* (New York: Cambridge University
Press, 1979), especially chs. 5, 6; and Jan Blanpain
*et al., National Health Insurance and Health Resources:
The European Experience* (Cambridge, Mass.: Harvard University Press, 1978). As Glaser notes, Germany is
unique in Europe in allowing "differences among funds
in benefits to the subscriber and in payments to doctors
for the same benefits" (p. 221). Even in the absence
of such competition, however, the funds' wish to assure
their mass membership that subscribers get a good value
for their money gives them an organizational incentive
to "represent the consumer" in bargaining with providers.

48. See Deborah Stone, "Health Care Cost Containment
in West Germany," *Journal of Health Policy, Politics,
and Law*, vol. 4 (1979), pp. 176-199. More generally,
see William A. Glaser, "Politics of Cost Containment
Abroad," *Bulletin of the New York Academy of Medicine*,
vol. 56 (1980), pp. 107-114.

49. Blanpain, *et al., National Health Insurance and
Health Resources*, pp. 41-42.

50. See Herman M. Somers and Anne R. Somers, *Doctors,
Patients, and Health Insurance* (Washington: The Brookings
Institution, 1961), chs. 14-16.

51. The phrase is taken from the title of Glaser's
recent book, cited in note 40 *supra*.

52. Glaser reports, for example, that: "The trend
in the world is toward collective regulation covering
entire provinces and entire countries . . ." and "to . . .
take many essential economic decisions out of the hands
of the parties to rate-setting of the individual hospital."
Centralization, he notes, is the French solution to
regulatory capture: "the financial ministries have the
final say, interministerial conferences keep everyone
busy preparing the guidelines, and the grassroots regulators are not consulted extensively by the key decision-
makers." William A. Glaser, "Paying the Hospital in
France," August 1980, pp. XIII-2, XIII-3, XIII-4.

53. Christa Altenstetter and James Warner Bjorkman, "Planning and Implementation: A Comparative Perspective on Health Policy," discussion paper series, International Institute of Management, Wissenschaftszentrum, Berlin, August 1979, p. 27.

54. A vignette from Great Britain may be pertinent. When the British Medical Association voted in July 1980 in favor of the abolition of community health councils, "watchdog committees set up in 1974 to represent consumers' interests in the health service," the chairman of the association general medical services committee argued that they should be retained. He was quoted as saying that ". . . when the Government is hell bent on cuts you need friends. Community health councils have probably done more to preserve local hospitals and local obstetric units than any other bodies." *The Times* (London), July 11, 1980.

55. William A. Glaser, "Paying the Hospital: Foreign Lessons for the United States (Some Preliminary Conclusions)," December 1979, pp. 6-7.

56. See Harvey M. Sapolsky, "The Political Sociology of Health Regulation," draft, January 1977, especially p. 2, and the essay in this volume. See also Mancur Olson, Jr., "The Optimal Allocation of Jurisdictional Responsibility: The Principle of 'Fiscal Equivalence'," in Subcommittee on Economy in Government of the Joint Economic Committee, *The Analysis and Evaluation of Public Expenditures: The PPB System,* 91 Cong. 2 sess. (GPO, 1969), vol. 1, pp. 321-331.

57. Klaus-Dirk Henke, "A Short Introduction into the German Health Insurance System," unpublished paper, p. 14, table 9.

58. According to Leichter: "The satisfaction and sense of pride expressed by the public, the apparently acceptable level of inequalities, and the generally high level of health and health care indicate that the system is working well. The problem of health care costs must be evaluated in terms of the questions: 'How much is the society willing to pay for health care?' Thus far, Germans and German policy makers appear to be willing to bear rather high costs." (*A Comparative Approach to Policy Analysis,* p. 154.)

59. Altenstetter and Bjorkman, "Planning and Implementation," pp. 38-39.

60. See Bovbjerg, "Problems and Prospects for Health Planning," pp. 93-97 *passim.*

61. Cain and Darling, "Health Planning in the United States," p. 15.

62. *Ibid.*

63. For a case in point, see Ely Devons, "The Problem of Co-ordination in Aircraft Production," in Alec Cairncross (ed.), *Papers on Planning and Economic Management by Ely Devons* (Manchester: Manchester University Press, 1970), pp. 37-58.

64. In the United States there are more abundant opportunities for influencing regulations and for exercising oversight over them than is often supposed. See Bruce C. Vladeck, "The Market vs. Regulation: The Case for Regulation," prepared for presentation at the Symposium on Health Care Regulation and Competition: Are They Compatible?, Project HOPE Institute for Health Policy Study, Millwood, Virginia, May 1980, especially pp. 18-20. Recent far-reaching discussions about, and changes in, the regulation of the airline, trucking, railroad, and telecommunication industries suggest that once agreement has been reached on the need for it, "reform" may come more quickly and easily than traditional capture and iron triangle theories maintain.

65. On the limits of formal coordination in the health efforts of one state, see Basil J. F. Mott, *Anatomy of a Coordinating Council* (Pittsburgh: University of Pittsburgh Press, 1968).

66. Mott, "The New Health Planning System," p. 245.

67. One of the more temperate accounts summarizes the issue in these terms: "Consider the 'highly technical' problem of evaluating the efficiency and effectiveness of sixty-one Detroit area hospitals in order to determine its bed reduction plan. Many of the proxy measures being used are automatically loaded in favor of the larger, tertiary care facilities, a seemingly technical decision with profound political overtones and possibly perilous consequences for access for the underserved." Consumer Coalition for Health, "Written Submission . . . ," pp. 2-3.

68. HSA participants sometimes complain of the other side of the coin: state CON staffs come under pressure from governors and legislators mobilized by provider interests and reverse tough HSA positions. Both patterns exist; it is now impossible to judge their relative frequency.

69. Edward C. Banfield and James Q. Wilson, *City Politics* (Cambridge, Mass.: Harvard University Press, 1963), ch. 14.

70. Herman Somers, *Presidential Agency: The Office of War Mobilization and Reconversion* (Cambridge, Mass.: Harvard University Press, 1950).

71. Robert Kagin, *Regulatory Justice* (New York: Russell Sage Foundation, 1978).

72. Lawrence D. Brown, "The Formulation of Federal Health Care Policy," *Bulletin of the New York Academy of Medicine,* vol. 54 (1978), pp. 45-58, especially pp. 56-58.

73. For instance, the head of New York City's HSA describes his agency as a means of providing alternatives to the efforts of public officials to "take drastic measures to shrink the health care system." The HSA, he believes, is "uniquely suited" to this task because its "orientation toward health and health planning enables us to avoid the danger of over emphasizing cost savings for their own sake." His HSA has taken "the bold and ambitious step of undertaking a series of related studies. . . ." Anthony L. Watson, "The View From the Health System Agency," *Bulletin of the New York Academy of Medicine,* vol. 56 (1980), pp. 55-57, quotations at pp. 56 and 57.

74. In the United States, the layers might be described as follows: (1) communitarian--decisions made in open, roundtable, town-meeting forums; (2) participatory--decisions made by a self-selected subset of activist community residents; (3) pluralist--decisions made by the interaction of local groups and organizations along with either of the two above modes; (4) corporatist--decisions made by organizations deliberately selected to represent major sectoral interests (along with any of the above three modes; (5) political-legal--decisions made by a subset of community residents formally chosen by election (along with the above four modes); (6) bureaucratic--decisions made by officials appointed by and accountable to political representatives; (7) federal--decisions made by interaction of some or all of the above processes between higher and lower levels of government. Decision-making might involve one, some, or all of these layers. Each has its distinctive strengths and weaknesses. The "optimal" representative layer or mix of layers for policymaking in a democracy is therefore a more complex question than much loose political theorizing about "participation" would suggest.

INTERSTATE VARIATION IN
CERTIFICATE OF NEED PROGRAMS:
A REVIEW AND PROSPECTUS*

Donald R. Cohodes

*Certificate-of-need and 1122 review of proposed capital
expenditures is considered by many to be the major
implementation tool of health planning. While, conceptually, capital expenditure review programs can be
used to further several planning goals, in practice, they
have been regarded as principally a tool for cost containment. In this paper, Cohodes describes variations
among CON programs and discusses reasons for such variations. He points up problems of CON program evaluations
and assesses the merits of various suggested program
changes.*

INTRODUCTION

State programs directed at controlling unnecessary or
duplicate hospital investment in plant and equipment
first surfaced in the 1960s. New York enacted the first
certificate-of-need (CON) law in 1964, followed by Rhode
Island (1968), Maryland (1968), Connecticut (1969), and
California (1969). In October 1972, Congress enacted

---

*Portions of this paper are based on a study conducted
by the author funded by the DHHS. The study was "Evaluation of the Effects of Certificate of Need Programs."
Contract number HRA-231-77-0114. The opinions expressed
in this paper represent those of the author and do not
necessarily represent those of the government.

P.L. 92-603, amending the Social Security Act. This act,
which reinforced state CON initiatives, stipulates that
federal funds under the Maternal and Child Health, Medicare, or Medicaid programs may not be used to support
"unnecessary capital expenditures made by or on behalf
of health care facilities or health maintenance which
are reimbursed under such programs." Implementation of
Section 1122 of P.L. 92-603 requires a plan for health
facilities and services review and a formal agreement
between the state and the federal government. The funds
to which Section 1122 refer are for interest, depreciation, or dividends from capital expenditures. States
participate in the program on a voluntary basis. The
Section 1122 review program differs in many ways from the
state-sponsored CON programs. The differences relate to
the sanctions that the programs can invoke, the contractual
linkage between the state and federal government, program
scope and procedures, and the appeals process.

A common misconception is that all state certificate-
of-need (CON) programs are the same. In fact, this is
hardly the case. State CON programs vary across a wide
spectrum; they have different coverage procedures, available resources, political support, application review
processes, and relationships with other organizations.[1]
In addition, the enthusiasm accompanying program implementation varies in conjunction with the state's
political regulatory milieu.[2]

Much of the discussion in this article is based on
the HRA-sponsored study, "Evaluation of the Effects of
Certificate of Need Programs." That study was a large
study employing a variety of analytical approaches and
a number of different data bases. The findings reported
in this paper are based on one component of the larger
research endeavor. The basic approach employed in the
reported study was a structured case study method.
Twelve states were selected for fieldwork, and site visits
were conducted. The principal exploratory information-
gathering technique employed in the study was a variation
of the tracer method. In each CON state visited, three
"interesting" cases of institutional interaction with
the CON program were examined. Through the investigation
and tracing of each case history, the larger picture of
the operation of the CON program was revealed. Interviews were conducted with an average of 20 individuals
in each of the 12 CON states and the 2 non-CON states.
These individuals included: CON program administration

and staff, state legislators or their staff, HSA and
SHPDA personnel, provider representatives, consumer
participants in the health planning process, other state
officials (e.g., rate-setting, licensure, or Medicaid),
representatives of third-party payers, individual physicians and hospital administrators, university observers,
and others. This broad range of interview subjects was
selected to ensure that all aspects of program operation
and interaction were considered. Structured discussion
guides were employed for each group of interview subjects
to ensure consistency of information collected across
states. In addition, formal detailed site visit reports
were prepared summarizing the information gathered in
each of the 14 site-visited states (12 with CON, 2
without).

The selection of the 14 study states was guided by
four considerations:

• the selection of a sample overrepresented in terms
of older CON programs,
• an appropriate balance of states with and without
hospital rate regulation and Section 1122 programs,
• a suitable geographic balance,
• the inclusion of non-CON states in the sample.

The 14 states selected and the year in which they
enacted CON were:

California--1969   Rhode Island--1968
Illinois--1974   South Carolina--1971
Maryland--1968   Texas--1975
Massachusetts--1971   Washington--1971
Minnesota--1971   Wisconsin--1977
New Jersey--1971   Louisiana--not enacted
North Dakota--1971   Pennsylvania--not enacted

Two other complementary activities were undertaken to
augment the case study fieldwork: document review and
file analysis and abstraction. For each state, state
health plans, health systems plans, CON legislation,
rules and regulations, special studies, etc., were reviewed and analyzed. Where appropriate, this material
was used to support and complement the information garnered
from the fieldwork. In addition to the document review
activities, individual CON program fields were abstracted
and relevant data on the CON review process was elicited.

In order to assess CON program performance it is
necessary to have a sense of the disparate environments
in which the programs operate. The role of a CON agency
may be very different in a state with an industry with
500 hospitals than a state with 25 hospitals. The
ability to monitor and understand hospital investment
plans decreases as the size of the industry increases.
When an industry attains a size of 100 to 150 hospitals,
it may result in a critical mass where problems in
reviewing and monitoring hospital investment plans begin
to grow geometrically. Table 1 provides a profile of
indicators of the variation in industry size and strength
in selected states. The variations are enormous. Hospital industry size ranges from 14 hospitals in Rhode
Island to 532 in California. Community hospital beds
per 1,000 population vary by 100 percent, and the role
of hospitals as key employers varies by as much as 65
percent. The point is simple: CON programs regulate
the investment behaviors of different hospital industries
and accordingly the problems in doing so vary by state.
    The fact that CON programs face a variety of problems
due to the size and structure of a state's hospital
industry is further complicated by the relative condition
of that industry. Two states may have similar-size
hospital industries, but one industry may be young with
few replacement needs, while the other may require massive
investment to bring it up to life safety code compliance.
While the data on asset vintage are limited, a 1975 PHS
study identified the percentage of beds found to be
nonconforming.[3] Even though it is not a direct measure
of asset age, the percentage of nonconforming beds can
be used as an alternative.* As an illustration, examine
Table 2. New Jersey and Washington have vastly different
renovation needs, but similar-size hospital industries,
New Jersey with 104 hospitals, Washington with 107. New
Jersey needs to upgrade 55 percent of its beds, while
Washington only has 9 percent of its beds out of compliance.

---

*Obviously, the percentage of nonconforming beds is an
inexact proxy for asset age. Unfortunately, good alternatives to it do not exist. Consequently, the reader should
be cautious in interpreting the measure as it is crude
and only provides a relative reference framework.

TABLE 1 Indicators of Industry Size and Strength (1976)--Selected States

State	Number of Community Hospitals	Number and Percent of Teaching Hospitals (Medical School Affiliation)	Community Hospital Beds per 1,000	Total Assets/ Community Hospital Beds (000's)	Employees as a Percent of All Nonagricultural Employees in the State
California	532	73 (13.7%)	3.75	62.6	2.60
Illinois	242	45 (18.6%)	4.87	63.4	3.30
Louisiana	134	19 (14.2%)	4.36	46.0	3.10
Maryland	50	22 (44.0%)	3.21	62.2	2.70
Massachusetts	117	38 (32.5%)	4.49	78.8	3.80
Minnesota	171	22 (12.9%)	5.92	46.5	3.21
New Jersey	104	28 (26.9%)	4.05	51.2	2.61
North Dakota	52	6 (11.5%)	6.42	41.6	3.70
Pennsylvania	246	64 (26.0%)	4.73	58.8	3.20
Rhode Island	14	8 (57.1%)	3.71	99.4	3.31
South Carolina	70	8 (11.4%)	3.69	38.7	2.30
Texas	495	34 (6.9%)	4.44	50.5	2.80
Washington	107	16 (15.0%)	3.24	66.2	2.31
Wisconsin	144	19 (13.2%)	5.23	47.2	3.11

SOURCE: Statistical Abstract, 1978, and *Trends in Hospital Construction*, ICF, Inc., 1978.

59

TABLE 2   Percent of Beds Evaluated as Nonconforming by State[a]

State	Percent of Beds Found Nonconforming (1975)	State	Percent of Beds Found Nonconforming (1975)
Alabama	5.5	Montana	40.7
Alaska	26.6	Nebraska	17.7
Arizona	11.3	Nevada	24.1
Arkansas	7.1	New Hampshire	27.7
California	15.1	New Jersey	54.9
Colorado	23.7	New Mexico	4.6
Connecticut	25.8	New York	29.8
Delaware	52.9	North Carolina	24.4
D.C.	12.6	North Dakota	13.7
Florida	10.0	Ohio	11.5
Georgia	12.3	Oklahoma	29.3
Hawaii	17.0	Oregon	13.2
Idaho	21.1	Pennsylvania	31.6
Illinois	15.8	Rhode Island	9.1
Indiana	25.8	South Carolina	16.8
Iowa	32.7	South Dakota	39.1
Kansas	31.9	Tennessee	17.5
Kentucky	15.5	Texas	21.1
Louisiana	26.2	Utah	18.6
Maine	33.0	Vermont	8.2
Maryland	12.1	Virginia	22.9
Massachusetts	37.4	Washington	8.9
Michigan	20.7	West Virginia	35.1
Minnesota	22.9	Wisconsin	19.9
Mississippi	6.4	Wyoming	8.6
Missouri	16.6		
		TOTAL	21.7

[a]Table 6, "Number of Beds Evaluated as Non-Conforming by State." Bureau of Health Planning and Resources Development, Division of Facilities Development, Health Resources Administration, Public Health Service, 1975.

In addition to industry characteristics, there are
other factors that influence the ability of the CON
agency to perform well. The particular form and scope
of CON legislation that evolves in a state represents
a product of the political dynamic resulting from the
interaction among legislators, governmental planners
and regulators, providers, insurance companies, and
consumers. Each party has specific goals and objectives
that it hopes to see realized through a CON program.
For example, the principal objective of state regulators
may be the minimization of cost increases in the hospital
sector, while providers may want to avoid the duplication
of services and prevent potential competitors from gaining access to their market. The balancing of these
different, and at times conflicting, objectives and the
relative political strength and sophistication of their
advocates has contributed to a lack of uniformity in
CON laws across states.

The variety of coalitions mustered to pass the various
CON statutes is also pertinent.[4] In Texas the threat of
possibly more stringent federal controls in the future
served as a stimulus for passage of CON. The Texas
hospital association, joining the administration's
effort, sought the legislation as a protective device
from destructive competition (in the sense of building
duplicative facilities). In Massachusetts and New
York, the governor and the legislature joined forces to
pursue CON legislation largely because of the growth
in the Medicaid budget.

The CON originating coalitions possessed varied goal
sets that have subsequently been reflected in the different pieces of state legislation. In North Dakota,
Illinois, Texas, and California, for example, access to
care is equally as important as cost containment. In
other states, the focus is on distribution; in still
others the major thrust is the elimination of duplication.[5] Not surprisingly then, the federal government,
with its principal focus on cost containment, finds
various state CON programs lacking. The pursuit of
these different goals sets, in all likelihood, will lead
to different outcomes. Judging CON programs by a sole
federal set of criteria when they are state programs with
varied goals is both nearsighted and unfair.

In perhaps a less visible, but nonetheless important
way, changes in political administration affect the vigor
of CON program implementation. To a large extent, interest

groups can influence the program's mandate as evidenced
in the legislative scope of coverage, program rules and
regulations, and the presence of loopholes, exemptions,
or grandfather provisions in the law. Changes in
political administration affect program implementation
and commitment more directly than program mandate. Program commitment or will is a necessary condition for
program success, though difficult to define in a quantitative manner.[1] It stands as a reflection of the commitment
to the program by a state's governor, the legislature,
and key program staff. Program will or commitment can
range along a continuum from industry restraint to protection of the status quo. The key to understanding
program commitment is frequently the agenda of the governor.
How important is the CON program? If it is perceived as
important, then financial and political resources will
be brought to bear on the program's behalf. As an
illustration, consider South Carolina.[4] South Carolina's
CON program has a comprehensive mandate, but it lacks
the support of the governor and, consequently, it tends
to flounder. On the other extreme there are programs
with a will but without a comprehensive mandate such as
California. In such a circumstance, program staff are
frustrated by legal constraints and cannot succeed because they have not been provided with the capacity to
do so (e.g., limited legislative scope).

DIMENSIONS OF CON PROGRAM VARIATION*

Because CON agency practices encompass a wide range of
technical, political, and legal activities, it is useful
to describe their variations along five dimensions:

    1. the level and use of agency resources;
    2. the development and use of resource criteria and
standards for project review;
    3. the conduct of the application review process;
    4. the use of bargaining and negotiation in decision-
making; and

------

*These five dimensions reflect characteristics of the
CON programs that have been hypothesized to relate to
program performance.

5. the organizational characteristics of the agency
and its relationships with other organizations and program
participants.

AGENCY RESOURCES

State agency resources are essential to the operation of
CON programs. Without adequate funds and staff, state
agencies are likely to encounter serious difficulties in
performing their mandated functions. In theory, agency
resource levels should be correlated with the anticipated
volume of CON applications processed in a given year.
Resource levels should also indirectly reflect the general
commitment of key state governmental officials to the
CON program. The observed variability in staff and budget
is displayed in Table 3. Not surprisingly, Table 3 reveals
large differences in staff, total budget, and application
volume by state.

In terms of relative annual expenditure per staff member, three programs in the sample deviate significantly
from the average of $24,500--Texas ($81,000 per capita),
California ($60,000), and Illinois ($49,000). These
three programs are the same three with the largest agency
budgets. The high per capita expenditures can most
probably be attributed to the legalistic nature of their
review processes.[1,5] Given the relative nonrestraining
record* of these states,[1] these numbers suggest that
high resource levels are not necessarily associated with
effective CON programs. In essence, resource levels only
represent the potential of a program to achieve its goals,
and, consequently, do not automatically ensure success.

Table 3 also reveals a number of other relevant observations. Most likely, the observed upper limit of the
average cost per application in Rhode Island ($7,050) and
North Dakota ($7,000) is a reflection of two factors:
(1) the small annual application volume of each program,
and (2) the fixed costs associated with maintaining a
CON staff. The variations in the ratio of applications
to review staff may also be a function of program peculiar-
ities. For instance, Minnesota's high 60:1 ratio is a

*Restraining refers to the orientation of the program and
a general focus on the restraint of industry growth.
Measures of restraint included cost and investment variables
as well as indicators of the process.

TABLE 3 CON Agency Resources in Selected States

State	Number of Applications Processed Annually (1978)	Annual Budget FY 1979 (000's)	Dollars per Capita Staff (000's)	Dollars per Application Processed	Total Number of Professional Staff	Number and Percent of Total Staff Devoted to Project Review	Ratio of Application to Review Staff
California	360	1,500	60	4,167	25	19 (76%)[a]	19:1[a]
Illinois	200	534	49	2,670	11	6 (55%)	33:1
Maryland	40	100	25	2,500	4	3 (75%)	13:1
Massachusetts	240	366	31	1,525	12	12 (100%)	20:1
Minnesota	60	24	24	400	1	1 (100%)	60:1
New Jersey	90	500	28	5,556	18	18 (100%)	5:1
North Dakota	25	175	29	7,000	6	3 (50%)	8:1
Rhode Island	20	141	35	7,050	4	4 (100%)	5:1
South Carolina	100	N.A.	N.A.	N.A.	6	5 (83%)	20:1
Texas	400	650	81	1,625	8	8 (100%)[a]	50:1[a]
Washington	120	156	26	1,300	6	6 (100%)	20:1
Wisconsin	210	325	22	1,548	15	7 (47%)	30:1

[a] In California, 6 of the 25 professional staff are attorneys. In Texas, 5 of the 8 staff are attorneys. However, since attorneys are integrally involved in project reviews, they are included in the table.

SOURCE: Policy Analysis, Inc., and Urban Systems Research and Engineering, Inc., *Evaluation of the Certificate of Need Programs*, HRA No. 230-7F-0165, Washington, D.C., Department of Health and Human Services, August 1980.

function of the program's decentralized review process
and reliance on the HSAs.

RESOURCE CRITERIA AND STANDARDS FOR PROJECT REVIEW

As the major policy instruments that define the bounds
of program discretion, resource criteria and standards
are influential in shaping CON program posture. The
presence of criteria and standards is not sufficient to
ensure proper follow through by the CON agency. Much
depends on the intrinsic nature of the criteria or
standards, including such factors as:[1,2]

1. Their basic orientation
    • general versus service-specific
    • formal versus informal
2. The relative emphasis placed on substance versus
procedure in the review.
3. The process employed in their development
    • internally (by CON agency staff) versus externally
    • with or without the aid of special committees/
       task forces containing recognized experts plus
       representatives of diverse groups
    • limited versus broad review and comment by
       outside groups (e.g., HSAs, providers, the state
       agencies, consumers)
4. Their application in project review
    • narrow versus broad interpretation by agency
       staff
    • strict versus inconsistent adherence to rules
       and regulations that govern their use.

Most, if not all, states have proposed criteria for
their program. Criteria are descriptive guidelines that
depict the fundamental areas of concern that must be
addressed in judging the merit of an application. They
are nonquantitative. In contrast, standards tend to be
highly quantitative and more explicit than guidelines.
Rather than merely stating (as criteria do) that a
demonstration of need is a necessary factor in project
review, standards prescribe how need will be met.
State variation in standard development and implementation is a function of many factors, which include: the
quality of agency leadership, the extent of executive
and legislative support, and the political strength and

will of providers and the agency's past track record.[6]
The relative balance of these forces is a factor in
determining whether standards are more substantive than
procedural and whether they are applied broadly or
narrowly.

Another factor that contributes to the relative
utility and quality of standards is the presence of a
good data base. Many HSAs and CON agencies lack the
information base necessary for the development of defensible standards. As a consequence, states that have
proceeded with the promulgation of detailed standards
have left themselves open to charges of capricious or
at best ill-advised action.

THE APPLICATION REVIEW PROCESS

A common misperception among many observers of the
regulatory process is that the CON application review
process is uniform among states. The available evidence
tends to contradict that belief.[1,2,15] The application
review process encompasses a good deal more than just
the physical review of a proposed project. In general,
the review process involves three distinct phases: the
preapplication consultation phase, the information
screening phase, and the analysis and review phase. Within each phase, states have developed rather distinct
approaches. In the first phase, contact between the
program and the prospective applicant usually involves
a mixture of: (1) technical assistance in the preparation
of the application, and (2) active negotiation regarding
the scope and projected cost of the proposed project.
Some states limit their preapplication consultation
activities solely to technical assistance, while others
concentrate their activities on modifying project scope
and cost. In addition, while HSAs normally take the
lead in preapplication negotiations, in some states,
notably Maryland and Illinois, the state also assumes
a large role.[4]

The second phase of the review process, information
screening, involves examination of the application for
completeness. This function is typically performed by
the staff of the state CON agency and of the HSA in
whose jurisdiction the proposed project falls. This
process is normally employed to fill in holes in the
applicant's proposal. However, in some states the

information screening phase is used as another opportunity
for the CON program to influence the content of submitted
applications before the start of full review and analysis.
This is accomplished through requests for additional information not required in the original submission and
through subtle prodding of the applicant during this
process.

The final phase of the application review process is
the analysis and review phase. States vary in the emphasis
placed upon various analytical tasks and responsibilities
during this phase. In particular, variation may be observed in:[1]

1. the quantitative nature of the state agency
analysis;

2. the form in which state agency staff present
findings to the chief decision-maker--formal recommendations versus summaries of fact;

3. the extent of shared review responsibilities with
other agencies
   - type of agency
   - area of analysis affected
   - the nature of the input: findings versus
     recommendation;

4. the relative analytic burden (state versus HSA); and

5. the locus of the burden of proof: program versus
applicant.

Following the review decision is a generally neglected
aspect of the CON process: project monitoring. Few
states actually follow projects once approval is granted.
Consequently, it is possible for hospitals to exceed
the scope of cost of the original application or possibly
build something other than what was initially stated (e.g.,
intensive care beds rather than general medical surgery
beds). Because of limited resources and the competing
demands of new applications, monitoring is generally
a low priority item for CON agencies.

BARGAINING AND FINALITY OF DECISIONS

Some have argued that regulation is a complex bargaining
process that evolves simultaneously from a number of
institutional arenas.[7] Advocates of this bargaining
model are most concerned with the implementation process,

that is, the process by which general statements of
governmental purpose of intent, normally stated in
enabling or authorizing legislation, are carried out.
It is argued that "Multiple interactions among the
regulated industry, the regulators, the underlying
technical character of what is being regulated, and the
larger social and political context do much to shape
the outcome of the bargaining. In particular, much
depends on who bears the costs and who has what resources
in the case of nonagreement. Yet, as in all bargaining,
outcomes are not perfectly determined. Instead, there
is much that regulators can do both in the short run
and in the longer run to alter outcomes and the context
that determines those outcomes."[7]

Bargaining is an essential and inherent component of
the CON review process. The whole process of application
submission is a dynamic one, in which the involved parties
engage in bargaining and negotiation on the various
specifications of the application. Bargaining takes place
at each stage of the application review process. Figure
1 graphically depicts this flow.

Different states have selected varied approaches to
bargaining. Some choose to become involved in bargaining
at every possible opportunity (e.g., Rhode Island),
while others generally eschew bargaining as a useful
tactic (Texas). In Rhode Island's case, the orientation
towards intensive bargaining is facilitated by the small
size of the state's hospital industry (14 hospitals). In
Texas, the emphasis on due process and procedure during
the application review process effectively precludes bargaining as a useful tactic.[4]

Bargaining and negotiation occurs during all phases of
the application submission and review process, although
the intensity with which it is pursued will vary by
review phase. Because few states have formal policies
with respect to bargaining posture, the tone and level of
negotiation is frequently dependent on the personalities
involved. This dependence on leadership and management
style contributes to a lack of homogeneity in bargaining
stances by state and HSA.

In most states, bargaining is not restricted to the
content of the submitted application (two exceptions are
Illinois and Wisconsin[4]). The major issues for bargaining
are normally the cost and scope of the project. However,
great variability exists among programs. For example,
Massachusetts emphasizes alternative approaches and

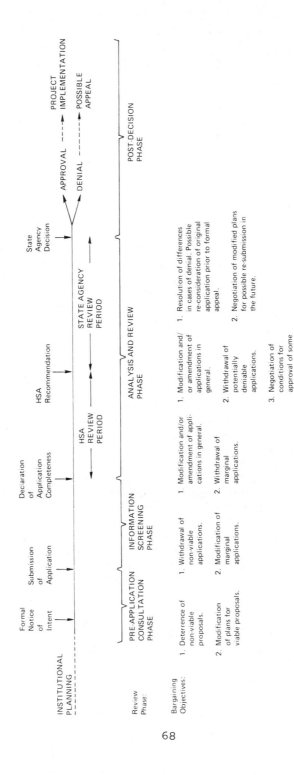

FIGURE 1 Bargaining and negotiation in the application review process.

services in addition to those discussed in the proposal. New Jersey discusses alternative financial mechanisms; North Dakota looks at timing effects on per diem costs, impact on related services, and referral arrangements; Rhode Island focuses on financing mechanisms and the potential for sharing services; and Texas treats time and space allowances.[4]

RELATIONSHIP WITH OTHER GROUPS AND ORGANIZATIONS

In sum, it appears that in context of application review, negotiations, and decision-making, the CON agency may become actively involved with a range of outside groups and organizations with interest in the regulatory process. In some cases, relations may take on a helpful or mutually supportive tenor. For example, relationships between the CON agency and local HSAs may prove very cordial if a particular state emphasizes the planning tool of CON review. However, in other states, the CON agency may have openly adversarial relationships with certain groups, thus compromising the potential for a productive working arrangement. Most group interactions are dependent upon the personalities and management style of the individuals involved in the review process. To the extent that these differ, organizational relationships will be affected.

Structural locations of the CON and related agencies also play a large role in determining mutual cooperation. For instance, in some states (e.g., Massachusetts) the CON agency is located within the health department laterally to the SHPDA. In other states (e.g., Rhode Island, Maryland, California, New Jersey) the CON agency is housed within the SHPDA, which is also located within the health department. In other states (e.g., Minnesota) the CON agency but not the SHPDA is located in the Department of Health. In still other states (e.g., Texas) the CON agency is an independent state commission. From the available data there is no apparent relationship between the location of the CON agency and its performance.

A variety of organizations and interest groups are involved in the CON review process. Table 4 displays these groups and the nature of the organizational relationships. The major observation that one takes from Table 4 is that CON interorganizational relationships are complex, diverse and vary by state.

TABLE 4 Organizational Location of CON Programs and Relationships with Other Organizations/Groups in Selected States

State	Organizational Location of Program	Organizational Relationships[a]					
		SHPDA Staff	Other State Agencies	HSAs	Groups	Governor	State Legislature
California	Health Dept.; in SHPDA	±	+	-	b	+	-
Illinois	Health Dept.; in SHPDA	±	Rate-setting: ± (developing)	±	Hosp. Assoc.: + Med. Assoc.: N	N	N
Maryland	Health Dept.; in SHPDA	±	Rate-setting: -	+	Hosp. Assoc.: + Blue Cross: + Med. Soc.: N	+	+
Massachusetts	Health Dept.; lateral to SHPDA	-	Rate-setting: +	+	b	±	-
Minnesota	Health Dept.; SHPDA not in Health Dept.	-	Rate review: +	++	Hosp. Assoc.: ±	+	+
New Jersey	Health Dept.; in SHPDA	+	Rate-setting: +	+	Hosp. Assoc.: + Blue Cross: + Med. Soc.: N	+	±
North Dakota	CON=SHPDA; in Health Dept.	++	+	±	Hosp. Assoc.: ++ Med. Soc.: +	N	N

State	Structural location		Rate regulation		Payer relations			
Rhode Island	Health Dept.; in SHPDA	+	Rate-setting: +	N.A.[c]	Blue Cross:	±	+	±
South Carolina	Health Dept.; in SHPDA	+	+	±	Hosp. Assoc.: + Med. Soc.: N	+	+
Texas	Independent State Commission	−	+	±	Hosp. Assoc.: ++ Med. Soc.: +	+	+
Washington	Deep within the Health Dept. and SHPDA	−	Rate-setting:++	+	Hosp. Assoc.: + Med. Soc.: −	N	N
Wisconsin	Health Dept. in SHPDA	−	Rate review: +	±	Hosp. Assoc.: + Med. Soc.: −	+	±

[a]Symbols indicate the following relationships:

++ = very close working relationship with frequent communication

+ = generally positive relations

± = relations vascillate from positive to negative at times

N = neutral relationship with little or no interaction

− = generally strained relations most of the time with little coordination or communication

−− = adversarial relationship.

[b]Adversarial relationship caused providers to seek exemptive legislation (Massachusetts) or to embark on court battles (California).

[c]Rhode Island has no HSA per se, but relations between the CON program and the Health Planning Council have been generally positive.

SOURCE: Policy Analysis, Inc., and Urban Systems Research and Engineering, Inc., *Evaluation of the Effects of Certificate of Need Programs*, HRA No. 230-7F-0165, Washington, D.C., Department of Health and Human Services, August 1980.

71

FACTORS AFFECTING PROGRAM SUCCESS

In the initial portions of this paper, evidence was presented on the state diversity of political, industry, and
CON program characteristics. Because of this lack of
homogeneity, it is difficult to identify those factors
that in all situations will be instrumental in assuring
better program performance. Still, there are some lessons
that can be gleaned from the review of state program
variation. Before discussing the set of factors that
can make a difference, it is important to set the context
in which CON programs operate.

First, although obvious, planning is an inherently
political and complex process.[8] From its inception, interest groups and political pressure have played a role in
shaping its structure and in influencing program implementation. Adding to this recognition of political reality
is the observation that CON programs operate under different program goal sets in different locales. Frequently,
this is a consequence of political pressures and the
relative strength of the affected provider industries.
Because state goals may be at variance with federal objectives, there often is a gap between program expectations
and program performance. This gap is exacerbated by the
differences in perceptions over the nature and extent of
the problem (e.g., one of distribution vs. duplication
of facilities) and the means available to do anything
about the problem. If the diagnosis of the problem in
a state concludes that insurance coverage is the culprit
behind hospital cost inflation, there is little, if
anything, that a CON program can do to rectify it. The
lack of consistency between perceptions and expectations
of the problem has been one factor leading evaluators to
sharply criticize the CON program. So long as evaluation
criteria different from state goals are employed to assess
program performance, judgments on CON's efficacy will continue to be harsh.*

---

*Even if goals are used as evaluation criteria, the assess-
ment of CON performance still may be harsh. The judgment
regarding which evaluation criterion to employ to assess
CON performance is still unsettled. Because the programs
have multiple goals, varied environments and resources,
different degrees of political support, and have paid
varied prices for passage, determining the set of performance criteria is a rather complex task. But, it is

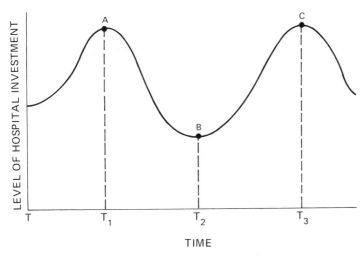

FIGURE 2   Illustrative investment cycle for a
state hospital industry.

There are two other factors that should be considered
when identifying elements that contribute to program
success. The first is time. Depending on the point
in time in the investment cycle of a state's hospital
industry a CON program comes on line, the program will
be perceived as successful or unsuccessful.[9] Figure 2
illustrates this point. If one assumes that hospital
investment follows a cyclical pattern,[9] then Figure 2
is a reasonable approximation of the ebb and flow of
investment. If a CON program is introduced at time T
and assessed during the interval T_2-T_1, it will appear
to be successful because the rate of hospital investment
declines from point A to point B. The fact that it does
so because of historical investment patterns and not
because of CON may be overlooked in a rush to declare the
program successful. On the other extreme, if a CON
program is introduced at time T_2 and evaluated during the
period T_3-T_2, it will appear to perform poorly because
hospital investment is on the rise. Again, the fact
that this may be occurring because of the historical

one that must begin with the recognition that while CON
programs share common characteristics, they are not homogeneous and they require detailed institutional understanding before a judgment on their performance can be rendered.

renovation needs of the industry may be overlooked and the CON program could be branded a failure, by capital restraint measures.

The second component of the time dimension is that there are considerable lags in time between the decision to invest and the completion of the observed physical structure. The implication is that the consequences of a CON decision in year one may not be observed until year 5, 6, or 7.[10] Evaluations of CON programs in their early life may inadvertently fail to attribute certain outcomes to the activities of the program.

The last consideration to bear in mind when assessing program performance is the political price necessary for passage. In many states, the price for passage of the CON statute was significant grandfather provisions, loopholes, or exemptions (see, for example, Texas, Illinois, and California's CON legislation). The consequences of this political price may be witnessed for a number of years after the time of program initiation. Not only will the performance of the agency be hindered by loopholes or exemptions, but staff morale and commitment also may be adversely affected.

DISTINGUISHING FACTORS

It can be argued that two conditions are necessary, though not sufficient, for program success: program mandate and program commitment or "will."[11] Program mandate refers to the legislative scope of coverage, program rules and regulations, and the presence of loopholes, exemptions, or grandfather provisions in the law. The federal government can take action to ensure that all states have the comprehensive mandate necessary to guarantee that the potential exists for successful program operation. This can be accomplished through the promulgation of national CON requirements for coverage, rules, and standards. Imbuing state agencies with the will or a commitment to restraining industry growth is a more challenging and less promising task. Commitment or will cannot be externally forced on a state agency or an HSA.

Program commitment or "will reflects the extent of executive support and the goal orientation of the CON agency staff. State agencies may vary from a purely process orientation to a more restraining stance, where the agency goal is to limit industry growth. Without a commitment to the restraint of industry growth, the most comprehensive, far-reaching program will likely fail to achieve its objectives. Similarly, even if the commitment to the restraint of industry growth is strong, the endeavors of the agency may be frustrated by legal constraints on authority.

If the federal government directly seeks to impose a mandate and will upon a recalcitrant state, the outcome, in terms of improved program performance, is likely to be negligible. Already states have pursued a variety of strategies to avoid the imposition of federal intervention (e.g., Utah's procompetitive CON statute).[12] The zeal with which a federally required program will be implemented also will depend on a state's agenda.[4] If a CON program and cost containment are relatively low on the governor's and the legislature's priority list, then it is safe to assume that program implementation will be less than enthusiastic. In order for a reluctant state to pursue a vigorous cost containment path, it is necessary that there be an incentive to do so. As presently constituted, failure to adopt a CON program theoretically could lead to substantial losses in public health service monies. However, these negative sanctions may prove politically difficult to use. Perhaps a better approach would consider the use of positive incentives. Such incentives might link the passage and effective implementation of a CON program to changes in revenue-sharing or increases in the federal share of Medicaid expenditures. Financial incentives of this nature could do much to encourage state commitment to the CON process.

An additional factor that distinguishes more successful CON programs is the presence of effective leaders and good managers. A recent study of the experience of 12 state CON programs points out that management can make a difference.[1] Good managers and leaders succeed in stretching the limits of their regulatory discretion. They are able to elicit loyalty and commitment to program goals from their staffs. Unfortunately, there is no magic formula that will produce gifted and competent managers and leaders. Financial incentives would help to attract managerial talent to a program, but that is not likely to be sufficient. Good managers and leaders will require executive support to effectively run their programs. A good manager can judge whether it is possible to achieve any improvement in program performance. If executive support is missing, attracting a competent manager will be a difficult task.

As mentioned earlier, the size and political potency of the provider industry will have much to do with the relative effectiveness of the CON program. A powerful,

well-organized, politically well-connected provider industry poses a different set of problems for a state CON
program than a fragmented, disorganized hospital industry.
Although the size and political clout of a hospital industry in a state are given, the selection of the strategies pursued to cope with the industry can be critical.

For hospital industries of less than say a hundred,
it should be possible to pursue individual negotiations
and cultivate valuable working arrangements. As industry
size grows, the feasibility of pursuing a negotiated
process with each hospital declines. When a CON agency
is confronted by a large, mature hospital industry (200
or more hospitals), with respect to agency resources, the
problems of monitoring and managing its activities can become overwhelming. In such a circumstance, it becomes
virtually impossible to pursue an individual institutional
dialogue. The CON agency then is faced with a number of
options:

1. it may try to conduct an individualized review and
be stretched thin;
2. it may rely on arbitrary mechanistic standards that
require little institutional analysis;
3. it may capitulate to the industry and seek to
take action on only the most flagrantly unnecessary projects; or
4. the agency may choose to streamline its review
procedure and concentrate on cost-effective reviews.

The first three alternatives are frequently observed and
to date have not yielded positive returns.[1,2] The fourth
option, of streamlining the review process, is potentially promising. It is discussed fully in the concluding
section.

In order to be successful, regulation requires that
regulators be skilled and allowed a modicum of discretion
where professional judgment can be exercised. The CON
programs have been characterized by a movement towards
greater specificity in the development and promulgation
of standards.[13] This movement has been encouraged by the
rapid legalization of the health planning process. In
some individual's eyes, P.L. 93-641 has become the
lawyers' equal opportunity employment act of 1975. The
emphasis on due process, procedure, and specificity is
a partial function of the enlarged legal presence. One
result has been the push for detailed standards. While

conceptually there is little wrong with detailed standards, in practical terms they pose problems. Their promulgation suggests a concreteness in the knowledge base that is missing. Moreover, detailed standards explicitly bind the discretion and latitude of a CON agency. Take for example the National Guidelines and the choice of point estimates, such as 4.0 beds/1,000, as a guideline. Had flexibility been built into the process with a range, e.g., 3.6 to 4.4 beds/1,000, instead of a point estimate, CON agencies would have been able to retain a certain discretion in their regulatory function without adversely affecting outcomes.* There is a danger in constraining CON activity through overly detailed standards. If discretion is completely removed, the CON process becomes nothing more than a procedurally explicit rubber stamp for proposed projects.

Obviously, there is a need for due process protection in the CON review--as there is a need for attorneys. The problem, however, is in striking the appropriate balance. At the moment the swing towards specificity may have gone too far. The reasons for this are complex, but stem from the belief that CON agencies are incompetent and not to be trusted with any discretionary authority. CON advocates, though, would argue that given the chance CON agencies would perform well. To date, the evidence available on the point is not sufficient to support or refute either contention.[14,15]

WHERE DO WE GO FROM HERE?

There are a number of directions that could be pursued in reforming or changing the CON process. The literature on the effectiveness of state CON programs strongly argues for changes in the programs if they are ever to be effective as cost containment mechanisms.[1,10,11,16,17] This section is divided into three components. The first contains a discussion of administratively simple and politically acceptable changes in CON programs. The second describes a set of proposed major changes. The last portion of this section describes the author's view of the likely prospects for the future.

---

*A certain flexibility already exists in the 4.0 beds/1,000 guideline as adjustments are allowed for such factors as age, population fluctuations, etc.

POLITICALLY ACCEPTABLE APPROACHES TO REFORM

There are a number of structural changes in the CON
program that could be accomplished with little political
opposition. One such change would be an improvement in
the agency's monitoring practices. At present, once
a CON is awarded, there is no formal mechanism in
place to ensure that what was proposed is what is actually
built.[11,13,18] Furthermore, there is no formal way to
guarantee that the original proposed costs remain as
final costs. Improving or instituting monitoring mechanisms would help to ensure that only a project's original
scope at the proposed cost is constructed. It is unlikely
that this type of change in the CON program would necessitate legislative action. In most states it could be implemented through administrative action, since monitoring
is normally included in a CON program's legislative
charge. In states where a rate-setting program is in
operation, the monitoring function could be accomplished
by the rate-setting authority without any necessary
changes in the CON program.*

A second change that is unlikely to stir the passions
of provider opposition would be the call for an improvement
in the quality of the data base used to reach CON decisions.
Currently, the absence of a good data base leaves the
CON agency open to charges of "blind budget-cutting without regard to quality or, alternately, of simplistic,
rigid planning evidenced by a mechanistic application of
formulas (for example, x number of open-heart surgical
procedures per year equals good care)."[13] In either
case, better data would provide CON agencies with an
improved potential to reach better decisions.

Another relatively innocuous reform that is likely
to be proposed is an increase in the available review
time. Presently, there is a great deal of variation in
the time alloted for state agency review of CON programs.
The range is on the order of 30 days (South Carolina) at
the low end to 240 days (Massachusetts) at the high end,
with most states providing 90 days.[1] Judging from the
experiences of those states who have had some success
with the CON program, a review period of approximately

---

*Public Law 96-79 now requires state programs to develop
effective monitoring procedures. Implementation of effective monitoring, though, is likely to vary by state.

120 to 150 days might be appropriate.[1] However, the actual desired review time is contingent on a number of factors: (1) the relative analytical burden assumed by the state and the HSAs, (2) the workload of the state agency staff, (3) the nature of the analysis required, (4) the extent of shared review responsibilities with other agencies, and (5) the relative preferences of program managers for quality versus efficiency in reviews. For example, if the staff workload is great and review requirements necessitate a sophisticated review, then to ensure a quality evaluation a longer review time would be required. Otherwise, if review efficiency is more important or if the staff workload is light, a shorter review period may be in order.

Another reform, which might be considered, is the requirement that every applicant engage in preapplication consultation.* Many planners believe that the scope and cost of a proposed project can be reduced through early and continued contact with the applicant. Frivolous projects can be discouraged at this point in the review process and a basis for future negotiations can be established.

A reform that has gained increasing attention and that has been required in the 1979 Health Planning Amendments is the notion of competitive reviews of CON applications.[19] Batching is the term used to describe this proposed method of processing CON applications. Application batching differs from the current means of processing applications in two critical ways: (1) it requires that applications be submitted and reviewed during a specific time period, rather than continuously throughout the year; and (2) it places a burden on the reviewing agency to determine the relative need for the proposed project. Batching, though promising in conception, may yield little in practice. There are very few categories of investment where hospitals directly compete. The one major exception is in the area of new technology. Here batching can help-- but batching will also be susceptible to political pressures. While projects may be rank-ordered, there is no assurance that all ranked projects from first to last will not be approved. Without a capital expenditure limit it is likely that batching will do little but add to the procedural complexity of the review process.

---

*Many states and HSAs are already engaged in extensive preapplication consultation.

The last reform normally mentioned in the literature[14] is the linkage of CON program review activities with rate-setting (where rate-setting authorities exist). Rate-setting authorities are able to look beyond the myopic capital cost focus of a CON agency and review the operating cost implications of a proposed project. By linking the cost review of the review process with the rate-setting authority, CON agencies should be able to strengthen their review of complex proposals. States have pursued very different strategies in linking their rate-setting and CON authorities. In Maryland, there is a creative tension between the Health Services Cost Review Commission (HSCRC) and the CON authority. In Maryland, the capital costs associated with CON approvals are not automatically passed through by the HSCRC. The HSCRC conducts their own review and has had a tendency to take a more stringent view than the CON agency. This relationship is in marked contrast to that witnessed in the state of Washington. In Washington, the Washington State Hospital Commission (WSHC) offers opinions, not recommendations, to the CON authority. Moreover, all capital costs associated with CON approvals are passed through by the WSHC.[26]

The various approaches discussed in this section will likely result in no more than marginal changes in CON program performance. Given the recent surge of critical literature on the program,[14,27] modest changes may not be enough to satisfy disgruntled critics. Major changes in the program may be required, either in terms of operation or with respect to objectives. In the next section, a number of proposed major changes in the CON program are discussed.

MAJOR CHANGES IN THE CON PROGRAM

Over the last 3 years,[20] there has been an increased clamor for major changes in the CON programs. The most frequently called for reform is the introduction of experimental capital "cap" programs.[2,3,11,13,15] The imposition of a cap on capital expenditures in a state would establish a fixed dollar amount that CON approvals could not exceed. The introduction of a cap would represent an open acknowledgement of the limitations of the CON process. The capital cap concept is based upon the premise that if a committed CON agency is given real power, it will perform well. While this is certainly possible, the evidence on CON performance[1,10,14] does not raise one's confidence in the agency's ability to run a capital cap program well.

There are many concerns that have been raised regarding
the introduction of a capital cap program. These concerns
include: the possibility of a long-term decline in the
condition of a state's hospital industry, the creation
of incentives for providers to low-ball project costs
at the front-end, the deterrence of hospital investment
in productivity enhancing projects,[3] and the nature of
the hospital response--shifts of investment into other
areas, leasing, contract for services, and so forth. A
recent study analyzing capital cap programs commissioned
by the National Center for Health Services Research reached
the following conclusions:[3]

1. If used by themselves, capital limit programs are
likely to require relatively stringent ceilings to achieve
a meaningful impact on operating costs.
2. Under each capital limit, the type of allocation
formula* had little impact on the overall operating costs,
but a measurable impact on the average condition of facilities and operating costs in individual states.
3. Even with a stringent ceiling and a desirable allocation formula, the impact of a capital investment limit
is quite sensitive to a range of local factors potentially
beyond DHHS control (e.g., the types of investment covered
under state CON laws, the ability of HSAs to estimate the
cost and quality effects of investments under comparison,
etc.).
4. Capital investment limits may improve the ability
of hospital rate regulators to control hospital costs.

As is clear from the ICF study and general skepticism
in the literature, there are serious concerns regarding
the potential effectiveness of capital limitation programs.
However, capital caps do offer the possibility of intro-
ducing direct limits on capital growth. Moreover, they
offer the possibility of shaping the nature of capital
investment and establishing relative priorities for the
future. Rather than rush headlong into a massive federal
program, it seems reasonable to have the federal government
provide support to those states that wish to pursue a
capital limitation strategy on their own. A series of
such "natural" experiments would provide the federal
government with the requisite technical, process information

---

*The study experimented with different limits and various
apportionment formulas.

needed to determine whether a national program should be considered. Such natural experiments would not, however, address the question of implementation in less hospitable environments.

The provision of aid to certain states represents a second major policy change. The first portion of this paper highlighted the variability in state environments and in program characteristics. The explicit recognition of this variability could be reflected in federal policy. Rather than seeking to bring all states up to some minimum level of compliance, resources could be targeted to certain key states that share the federal government's goal set. Persuading Louisiana to introduce and implement a vigorous CON program, when it is not desired, is a fundamentally futile endeavor. Providing New Jersey, New York, or Michigan financial and technical assistance to pursue and expand their programs is an investment that at least has the potential to yield a return. In essence, the federal government should consider providing aid, in the form of ongoing or demonstration grants, to those states that are already actively pursuing cost containment strategies. Spending money on states that do not have a commitment to the CON process is equivalent to throwing good money after bad. A policy of concentrating on certain key states also may yield dividends nationally. By focusing on 10 to 15 key states, states in which perhaps 60 percent of all hospital resources are located, cost containment efforts could produce sizable returns.*

A third major change in the CON process would approach the problem of excess capital investment from a slightly different perspective. This approach, aptly named the capital strangulation program,[21] has received heightened attention lately.[22] Basically, the approach entails limiting government-sponsored hospital investment subsidies and hospital access to debt. The first iteration of this strangulation strategy has surfaced in two hospital con- struction policy memorandums to the President. The mem- orandums call for a new project review process that "would specify that all new federal loans, loan guarantees, grants, and tax subsidies will require prior approval by the state and local planning process in the context of an

---

*There are 12 states responsible for more than one half of all hospital costs. They are: California, Illinois, Pennsylvania, Ohio, Texas, Michigan, Florida, Missouri, Tennessee, Georgia, North Carolina, and New York.

approved state and local bed reduction plan."[22]   The thrust
of this approach is relatively straightforward: first, it
makes federal investment subsidies or the allocation of
capital funds consistent with other policies (e.g., cost
containment), and secondly, it effectively raises the
price and limits the availability of capital.   The
coordination of government subsidy and debt programs
with CON programs would add another policy lever that
could be used to influence the mix and quantity of
hospital investment.

The implementation of a policy such as this is fraught
with difficulty and may be subject to intense policy
opposition (e.g., special interest groups such as the
Veterans Administration).   The effectiveness of this
policy may be limited to major capital projects as alternative financing sources to the government can be located
for small purchases.   Moreover, if hospitals are forced
to seek out alternative, more costly financing, total
project costs may be higher than they would have been
with government financing.

A fourth potential change would not directly involve
the CON agency, as it would be directed at third-party
payors and rate-setting authorities.   This policy would
necessitate alterations of hospital capital cost reimbursement.   Hospitals obtain funds for investment purposes
from internal and external sources.   Rate-setting authorities and third-party payors are in a position to establish policies that would limit the flow of capital into
the hospital sector.   Policies regarding the treatment
of the recovery of depreciation, net revenues, and debt
can serve to restrain or encourage capital formation.
There are many ways in which this can be accomplished.
For example: replacing the present capital cost reimbursement with an all-inclusive capital charge allowance built
into hospital rates, or establishing a ceiling on total
capital cost reimbursements, or reimbursing actual interest
expenses up to a maximum effective interest rate.   In addition to modifying capital cost reimbursement policies,
it is also possible to modify reimbursement of operating
costs.   One result would be a squeeze on hospital net
revenues and the placing of pressure on inefficiently
utilized capacity.   Possible approaches to changing
operating cost policies include: reimbursing operating
costs on the basis of fixed prices for individual services,
or a fixed total per day or per patient or on the basis
of the type of illness treated, and adjusting reimbursement rates to reflect overall hospital efficiency.[23]

The consequences of pursuing this strategy are mixed for a CON agency. While on one hand, hospital investment plans will be influenced by altering capital and operating reimbursement policies, the CON agency will be dependent on third-party payors and rate-setting authorities for the implementation and operation of the policy. Although attractive theoretically, the practical matters of "policy turf" may stand as a serious impediment to the success of this strategy.

PROSPECTS FOR THE FUTURE

Over the next 5 years, it is highly likely that in many states the CON program will undergo some major changes. Although some of CON's critics have called for its demise, that prospect seems unlikely. CON programs have developed their own constituencies, and, in conjunction with their reputed incompetency, it is highly improbable that there will be a widespread provider-sponsored call for their removal. In all likelihood there will be a subtle shift in cost containment strategies at the state level. CON programs will remain, but the key decisions will become the responsibility of the rate-setting authority. This switch in the locus of decision-making for capital project reviews has already begun in some states. In Maryland and Rhode Island,[24] the rate-setting authorities have extended their involvement in reviewing proposed capital projects. Yet, in spite of the conceptual appeal of increased rate-setting responsibilities regarding capital, few states have exhibited a great deal of enthusiasm for embracing rate-setting authorities. This may change as a number of recent studies have highlighted the effectiveness of these agencies.[27,28,29]

One prospect for the future of state CON programs is an increase in the size of the agency's legal staff.[13] An inevitable by-product of regulatory maturity and a result of the provider-generated demand for program specificity will be increased litigation. Already serious legal concerns over the planning law have surfaced, the most notable being the Justice Department's "business review," which raised the possibility that certain planning activities may violate antitrust laws.[22] The prospects for the future of the health planning process most certainly include increases in the level of litigation.

One of the most appealing CON reforms that may be
acted upon has been proposed by Schneider[25] and Bromberg.[12]
Both authors call for a major change in the CON review
process. Schneider's study of New York State's CON program demonstrates "that capital expenditures are minor in
comparison to operating expenditures and that the relationship between the two varies substantially depending on
the type of investment."[25] Based on this result, major
policy revisions are recommended for the CON program.
These are:

1. CON should seek to control access and availability
of patient services, not health care capital.
2. CON should focus on patient care programs, which
are the most costly elements of the system. Control of
other investments should not be included in the CON
system.
3. CON should expand the review to include the full
cost of health services, not only the capital cost.
Further, the review should be a cost-effectiveness review.
4. Decision-making authority for most capital investments, excluding those noted in (2), should rest with the
provider.
5. Economic incentives/penalties to control unnecessary capital investments, for those areas in (2) ceded to
the providers, should be developed within the reimbursement system.[25]

This approach seeks to introduce cost-effective reviews
into the CON system. Under this strategy, only patient
care service projects, selected high-technology areas,
and other big-ticket items would be subject to an intensive review. The system proposed would, to a certain
extent, deregulate the CON process. It would leave many
investment options in the domain of the provider and
seek to influence those decisions through financial incentives. The reforms proposed are predicated on the
functioning of an active and aggressive rate-setting
authority. In Schneider's words, "The system requires
that internal capital investment decisions, which are
decontrolled on CON, be implicitly controlled through
reimbursement."[25]
The benefits of this approach are many. They include:
(1) the reduction of government intervention in the internal investment decisions of hospitals, (2) a refocusing
of CON on those areas that have the greatest cost impact,

and (3) an expanded review of project cost implications--
capital and operating. Moreover, given the current de-
regulation mood in the Congress and in the state legislatures, a proposal to reduce the scope of CON's coverage,
rely more on financial incentives, and concentrate on
cost-effectiveness issues is bound to be appealing.

Finally, it is likely that the future will find increased flexibility in the application of standards in
various locales. This flexibility may be coupled with
targeted programs of financial and technical assistance.
One possibility would be a more explicit linkage of the
health planning guidelines to reimbursement systems.
Where reimbursement is cost-based and retrospective, the
current guidelines may be relevant. Where reimbursement
is prospective and based on efficient hospital behavior,
different incentives are at work, and waivers of the
guidelines may be in order.

In all likelihood, CON will begin to focus more on
planning and access issues than on financing issues.
This deemphasis of CON as a cost containment mechanism
will likely be accompanied by an increased reliance on
financial incentives generated by the reimbursement
system. While there will be a role for CON, it will be
one of reduced dimension and limited focus with the rate-
setting authorities moving to the forefront in the effort
to contain health care costs.

REFERENCES

1. Policy Analysis, Inc., and Urban Systems Research
and Engineering, Inc., *Evaluation of the Effects of
Certificate of Need Programs,* HRA No. 230-7F-0165, Washington, D.C., Department of Health and Human Services,
August 1980.

2. Codman Research Group, *Final Report: Health Planning and Regulation: The New England Experience,* HEW No.
291-76-0003, Washington, D.C., DHHS, September 30, 1979.

3. ICF, Inc., *An Analysis of Programs to Limit Hospital
Capital Expenditures,* Contract No. 233-79-3002, Washington, D.C., DHHS, June 30, 1980.

4. Urban Systems Research and Engineering, Inc.,
Twelve Case Studies of Certificate of Need Programs, HRA
No. 230-7F-0165, Washington, D.C., DHHS, August 1980.

5. Chayet and Sonnenreich, P. C., *Certificate of Need:
An Expanding Regulatory Concept,* Washington, D.C., 1978.

6. D. Altman and H. M. Sapolsky, "Writing the Regulations for Health," *Policy Sciences* 7, 1976.

7. P. Feldman and M. Roberts, "Magic Bullet or Seven Card Stud," Harvard School of Public Health, Boston, 1978.

8. T. R. Marmor, D. Wittman, and T. Heagy, "Politics, Public Policy, and Medical Inflation." Eidted by Michael Zubkoff, in *Health: A Victim or Cause of Inflation,* New York, Milbank Memorial Fund, 1976.

9. J. Howell, personal communication based upon unpublished doctoral dissertation at JFK School of Government, Harvard University, June 1980.

10. F. A. Sloan and B. Steinwald, "Effects of Regulation on Hospital Costs and Input Use," Proceedings of the 1978 Annual Meeting of the American Economics Association, Chicago, 1978.

11. D. R. Cohodes, *Institutional Response to Regulation: Certificate of Need and Hospitals,* doctoral dissertation, School of Public Health, Harvard University, Boston, January 1980.

12. M. D. Bromberg, "Health Planning and Certification of Need: Can Protectionism be Justified?" presented at the Project Hope Symposium on Competition and Regulation, May 22-25, 1980, Federation of American Hospitals, Washington, D.C., 1980.

13. M. K. Schonbrun, "Making Certificate of Need Work," *North Carolina Law Review* 57(6), August 1979.

14. D. R. Cohodes, C. Cerf, and J. Cromwell, *Certificate of Need Programs: A Review, Analysis and Annotated Bibliography of the Research Literature,* Washington, D.C., DHHS, 1978.

15. R. Bovbjerg, "Problems and Prospects for Health Planning," *Utah Law Review* 1978 (1).

16. G. Melnick, "Effects of Regulation on Hospitals," thesis in progress, University of Michigan, Ann Arbor, 1980.

17. D. S. Salkever and T. W. Bice, *Impact of State Certificate of Need Laws on Health Care Costs and Utilization,* Washington, D.C., U.S. DHEW, 1976.

18. W. Bicknell and D. C. Walsh, "Critical Experiences in Organizing and Administering a State Certificate of Need Program," *Public Health Reports,* January-February 1976.

19. Public Law 96-79.

20. Title II of the Hospital Cost Containment Act of 1977, H.R. 6575.

21. H. M. Sapolsky, "Capital Ideas: Options for the Control of Capital in the Health Sector," MIT, Cambridge, 1979.

22. "The Blue Sheet," *Drug Research Reports,* May 28, 1980.

23. ICF, Inc., NCHSR, Contract No. 233-79-3002, November 1979.

24. D. R. Cohodes, "The State Experience with Capital Management and Capital Expenditure Review Programs," Bureau of Health Facilities, HRA, February 1980.

25. D. Schneider *et al., Economic Impact and Project Selection Methodology for Certificate of Need,* New York State Health Planning Commission, May 1980.

26. D. Hamilton (ed.), "Rate Regulations," *Topics in Health Care Financing* 6(1), Fall 1979.

27. B. Steinwald and F. Sloan, "Regulatory Approaches to Hospital Cost Containment--A Synthesis of the Empirical Evidence," presented at an American Enterprise Institute Conference on Health Care in Washington, D.C., September 25, 1980.

28. General Accounting Office, "Rising Hospital Costs Can Be Restrained by Regulating Payments and Improving Management," September 19, 1980.

29. B. Biles, C. Schramm, and J. G. Atkinson, "Hospital Cost Inflation Under State Rate-Setting Programs," *New England Journal of Medicine* 303:664-668, September 18, 1980.

MONITORING THE HEALTH PLANNING SYSTEM: DATA, MEASUREMENT AND INFERENCE PROBLEMS

George W. Downs

*Questions concerning the impact and effectiveness of the
planning program are being posed in increasing numbers.
The future shape of planning, and even its continued
existence, may rest on the answers to these questions.
In the following paper George Downs highlights some
technical and conceptual problems of measuring planning
effects and suggests approaches which may, at least, miti-
gate the impact of these problems. His comments on the
proper design of experiments should be of interest to those
seriously considering evaluating the planning program.*

The most frustrating aspect of public life is not
the inability to convince others of the merits of
a cherished project or policy. Rather, it is the
endless hours spent on policy discussions in which
the irrelevant issues have not been separated from
the relevant, in which ascertainable facts and relationships have not been investigated but are the
subject of heated debate, in which considerations
of alternatives is impossible because only one proposal has been developed, and, above all, discussions in which nobility of aim is presumed to
determine effectiveness of program.--Charles L.
Schultze (1968:75)

INTRODUCTION

At the present time there are substantial gaps and uncer-
tainties in the knowledge-base that guides the formation

89

of health care policy. On the most fundamental level,
the benefits and costs associated with medical care
practices ranging from various surgical procedures to
the organization of emergency services are constantly
being revised in light of new research. As we move away
from basic services to broader issues involving alternative modes of financing and quality control, the gaps become even larger. Relevant supply and production functions
remain unspecified, and the ability of policymakers to
anticipate the response of doctors, hospital administrators, insurers, and consumers to various regulatory
initiatives and incentive schemes is marginal at best
(Berry, 1978).

Much also remains to be learned about how and how
well the planning and regulatory apparatus established
by the 1974 National Health Planning and Resources
Development Act (P.L. 93-641) and subsequent amendments
is working. To precisely what extent have health services
been "better" allocated and costs reduced below what they
otherwise would have been during the past 6 years? Have
some Health Systems Agencies (HSAs) been more successful
than others in accomplishing their mandated goals? If so,
does the explanation lie in the size and quality of their
staffs, their access to information, the priorities of
their board members, the nature of their relationship with
other agencies, or elsewhere? How critical is the development of quantitative, service specific standards to the
operation of an effective certificate-of-need program?
In short, what can the experiences of P.L. 93-641 agencies
tell us about the best way to control health care costs,
ensure access to care, and increase service delivery
quality?

What follows is an attempt to describe quite generally
some of the barriers that stand in the way of answering
such questions and impede the development of a satisfactory
"technology" of planning and regulation. The first section
contains a description of the barriers and a discussion
of why they exist. In the second section, a number of
research prescriptions are offered that might be employed
to help overcome them. No special claim is made about
the originality of these prescriptions. In each case,
their inclusion has been motivated less by their novelty
than by their importance and the extent to which they are
consistently disregarded.

PART I: PROBLEMS, PROBLEMS

Measuring the Impact of Planning and Regulation

A major problem with impact assessment in this area is
the sheer magnitude of the task. Health planning agencies
are operating under an exceedingly broad mandate. The
responsibilities assigned them under P.L. 93-641 include
restraining cost increases, improving the general health
status of the population, and increasing the accessibility, continuity, and quality of care. Competently
monitoring the achievement of these goals requires the
development of literally dozens of "performance measures"
and the collection of large amounts of reliable data.
Neither is easy, both are expensive.

Our present inability to predict the full consequences
of planning and regulatory decisions increases this burden
still further. Unanticipated consequences and spillover
effects inevitably accompany broad policy decisions and
they must be detected. This seems like an elementary
point, but its implications are rarely appreciated. Far
too much time has been spent in debating the goals of
health planning as a prelude to establishing data collection
procedures and reporting requirements. Data collection
cannot be restricted to narrowly defined "goals." One
must not, as Schweitzer (1978:73) argues, "fall into the
trap of measuring the success of a regulatory program
tautologically by measuring only what is directly regulated
while other objectives escape attention and are allowed
to get out of control." It was not one of the goals of
early certificate-of-need (CON) and rate-setting programs
to inspire the expansion and new construction of private,
physician-owned diagnostic and treatment facilities, yet
if empirically substantiated it is a consequence of some
significance. Similarly, if reducing capital expenditures
for long-term care facilities results in increased lengths
of stay in hospitals or if a rate structure designed to
penalize low medical/surgical bed occupancy stimulates
unnecessary elective surgery (Bauer, 1978:27), these effects
must be uncovered before any final judgment about the worth
of the program is made.

Selecting summary measures of health system resources
and performance that can serve as bases for policymaking
is also a problem. A given number of beds per 1,000 does
not represent the same thing in a rural area with low
population density as it does in the central city. Those

responsible for establishing desirable bed-to-population ratios are fully aware of this and set the target somewhat higher for rural areas. Other standards are vulnerable to similar but less obvious problems. A recent article by Sterman and Schaumberg (1980) on the use of the CT scan suggests that a reliance on number of scanners per 1,000 population as the principal basis for CON decisions could have a number of unfortunate consequences. Access opportunities to scanners in doctors' offices and small clinics vary substantially across income groups, and the authors note that in some areas many such units had been installed while municipal hospitals were still without them. In addition, the contribution that scan data made to arriving at a final diagnosis was found to be considerably greater in municipal hospitals than in private facilities, presumably because the former deal with patients who are more ill. Thus an apparently uniform standard might have dramatically different access and quality-of-care implications in suburbs and cities.

The data-gathering and analytic demands surrounding output and outcome measures are further exacerbated by the inferential limitations of most nonexperimental policy evaluation. Linkages between characteristics ·of planning agencies, their decisions, and health service and health status outcomes are notoriously difficult to establish. This is due in large part to the limited statistical ability to control for the effects of numerous potential sources of variance. The difficulties that this problem poses are common in health care evaluation. Municipal hospitals have, for example, always objected to the use of crude mortality rates as an indicator of quality of care because those rates can be dramatically affected by variables that lie outside their control (e.g., patient condition at time of admission). They argue that private hospitals will appear to be more effective simply because they deal with a different mix of patients.

An obvious solution to this problem is to statistically control for variables such as patient condition at admission, age, sex, medical history, and so forth. However, there are limits to how many variables can be controlled. When the number of such intervening and confounding variables is large and substantial multicollinearity is present, it may be necessary to choose another quality-of-care measure that is less vulnerable to extraneous factors. As McAuliffe (1979) has recently noted, the most viable alternative often appears to be a measure that focuses on the process of care (what is done) rather than on the outcome. In the case of hospital care, we might look at the process of diagnosis or infection rates under the assumption that variation in these indicators is more directly under the control of service delivery institutions.

The same logic holds when one is attempting to assess the impact of planning (or regulation). Health status outcomes such as morbidity and mortality rates are vulnerable to a variety of external sources of variation, many of which are not well understood. Unfortunately, some of the most commonly scrutinized health system "process" measures, particularly those associated with cost of care, are as subject to the effect of external factors as are health status outcomes. As we shall see, apart from relying more heavily on carefully designed policy experiments, the best way to deal with this problem is to further expand the list of process measures to include those that are subject to the direct control of planning agencies.

Discovering What Matters and How Much

The list of process and outcome measures that warrant attention is intimidating, but it pales in comparison with the list of health system and environmental variables that we have reason to believe have a significant impact on those measures. The reasons for this extraordinary number of potentially important determinants--even by the standards of those analysts exploring the sources of outcome variation in education or corrections--lie in: (1) the decentralized and pluralistic nature of the health planning system; (2) the limited amount of positive regulatory control vested in HSAs, Statewide Health Coordinating Councils (SHCCs), and State Health Planning and Development Agencies (SHPDAs); and (3) in the latitude that is permitted these agencies in implementing and supplementing the provisions of P.L. 93-641. In a very real sense, the design of the present planning and regulating system not only restricts what can be done, but it also greatly restricts our ability to accurately assess what it is doing.

The decentralization that characterizes the present health planning system makes it necessary to construct variables that can capture the priorities that are pursued

at the local level. Within broad outlines, HSA priorities
are locally established not federally mandated and they
vary substantially across the country. These priorities
have a direct impact on decision-making and probably influence the effect of numerous other variables as well
(e.g., the impact of HSA staff expertise in cost
accounting on CON decisions is likely to depend on the
priority the board places on limiting capital spending).
The pluralistic participation and decision structure
raises the additional prospect that any number of organizations or individuals can have a substantial influence on
key decisions. Hence the activities and resources of
legislators, consumer groups, hospital associations, and
medical groups, etc., are all potential determinants.

The 1974 National Health Planning and Development
Act represented an unprecedented merger of planning and
regulation, but the regulatory powers that it granted
were modest. While certificate-of-need programs
were mandated and state-local input solicited through
1122 contract recommendations, certain omissions are
just as noteworthy. The law, as Bauer (1978:28) nicely
summarizes, provides:

> no budgetary framework or annual caps on health
> expenditures within which planners could spell
> out priorities, or within which reviewers could
> reach decisions on institutional expansion, or
> definitions of "appropriateness";
>
> no way to fund start-up and operating costs of
> alternatives to inpatient care and prevention
> programs, or to pay the closeout costs of un-
> needed facilities;
>
> no power to influence where physicians practice,
> their referral networks, their staff privileges
> or their degree of cost consciousness when or-
> dering ancillary services;
>
> no power to prevent non-institution based
> physicians or others from acquiring facilities
> and equipment that, for institutions, would be
> subject to certificate of need regulations;
>
> no power to influence the many federal, state,
> and local regulatory bodies and voluntary agen-
> cies whose decisions may push up institutional
> costs;

no authority to bring federal hospitals under the
aegis of local and state planning and regulation.

As a result, the different components of the health
planning system collectively represent a highly constrained
regulatory authority that is virtually powerless to cancel
out the effect of exogenous shocks to the health care
system. Because such shocks can be produced by any number
of sources,[1] the list of potentially important determinants
is dramatically increased over that which might be associated with a strong regulatory authority.

This same limited regulatory authority has also created
a situation in which much of the effectiveness of HSAs
appears to depend on their timing, bargaining ability,
and what is often referred to as "political sophistication."
Every detailed examination of CON operation or P.L. 93-641
implementation has stressed the importance of these
"strategic" variables. Apart from increasing the number
of variables that we have to think about, these additional
factors pose difficult measurement problems. It is considerably easier to devise measures capable of capturing
the ability of HSAs and SHPDAs to process complex technical and accounting data than to measure their ability
to establish satisfactory liaison with PSROs or conduct
delicate negotiations with hospital boards.

The latitude permitted states in implementing and
supplementing the basic provisions of P.L. 93-641 also
increases the number of potential determinants. The formal
organizational relationships among relevant agencies, the
extent to which different consumer interests are actively
represented in HSA and CON laws, all vary substantially
from state to state. Certificate-of-need laws present
a typical case: they differ in their scope of coverage,
exemptions and grandfather clauses, nature of the appeals
process, and the range of sanctions that can be applied.
Each of these differences represents a possible source of
outcome variation.

The multiplicity of potential determinants poses
several difficulties for researchers. First, it is not
possible to analyze the impact of one variable (e.g.,
strength of CON law, or HSA board composition) in isolation.
If the analyst ignores other important independent variables, the variation associated with them is included in
the residual standard deviation, which is therefore much
increased. This shrinks t scores and results in insensitive tests for significance. Furthermore, when independent

variables are correlated (as they inevitably will be in observational studies), the size and even the sign of the coefficient may be different when estimated by itself as compared to its estimate in the presence of other determinants. There is no escaping the fact that the generation of accurate inferences will necessitate collecting a great deal of data and elaborate, multivariant analysis.

Second, the likelihood that many factors will influence the outcomes of interest (e.g., cost, access patterns, etc.) makes program evaluation difficult. The determination of what a given program or policy has accomplished must be based on some estimate of what would have occurred without it. To evaluate a CON program we need to know what capital expenditures would have been had no CON program existed. In an experiment this estimate is provided by a control group, but in a quasi-experimental setting it must be generated by some model. Everything else being equal, the more variables there are to contend with, the more difficult it will be to create a model that can provide this "counterfactual" forecast to use as a basis for judging program success.

Third, there is the problem of multiple comparisons. If the analyst begins with 20 or 30 potentially important determinants and reduces this number substantially by stepwise regression or a similar technique, the t scores and R-squared values are greatly inflated due to selection. Because t scores are random quantities that may be larger or smaller than true values, some percentage (e.g., 5 percent) of variables will appear significant when, in reality, they are not. The more variables that are employed in the analysis, the more likely it is that some that have no effect will be included in the final model.

Finally, there is a fourth problem that is behavioral rather than statistical. When the pool of prospective determinants is large, the careful consideration of all possible relationships is both bothersome and time-consuming. A rare amount of self-discipline is required to avoid the careless elimination of variables for reasons of convenience or as a consequence of the insensitive application of a dimension-reducing technique such as factor analysis. However, while it is true that a 25-variable model that purports to account for interstate capital spending variation would be absurd from the standpoint of estimation, the adoption of strictly mechanical methods of data analysis (in either a hardware or analytic sense) generally produces worthless results.

Coping with Interaction

A large number of potentially important variables is only one aspect of the complexity encountered by the quantitative researcher in this area. Another is the prevalence of interaction. To state that there is interaction between two variables is, of course, to say nothing more than that the impact of each depends on the magnitude of the other. Boyle's law, for example, tells us that pressure and temperature have an interactive impact upon the volume of a gas. The effect of a 1° increase in temperature depends on the amount of pressure that exists. Similarly, recent research on the effect of exercise on heart disease indicates that it depends on the kind of exercise, the physiological condition of the subject, and a number of environmental factors. Increasing exercise has no single, easily specifiable "impact" on vulnerability to heart disease; rather it has a variety of contingent effects, none of which is more fundamental than any other.

To fully appreciate the problem that excessive interaction poses in general, it is useful to consider the following dilemma described by Cronbach (1976). It appears that to predict a subject's voluntary delay of gratification, one must know the subject's age, sex, the models to which he or she was just exposed, the particular objects for which he or she is waiting, his or her immediate prior experience, and certain characteristics of the experimentor. By itself this is commonplace; most behaviors are multicausal, and this list of variables is relatively modest in length. The novelty (and horror) of the situation lies in the evidence, which indicates that the impact of any of these variables depends on *at least* four others. This makes statements about relative impacts out of the question and the formulation of a reasonably predictive model is difficult if not impossible.

Talk about interaction effects should not be dismissed as an exercise in methodological aesthetics. Their importance has long been appreciated by biostatisticians and clinical researchers through whose work they have had an important influence on public health recommendations. Consider the following predictive equation (adapted from Hammond, 1979):

$$\hat{Y} = 11.3 + 47.1X_1 + 111.3X_2 + 431.9X_1X_2.$$

Here Y = age-adjusted cancer death rate/100,000; X_1 = indicator for exposure to asbestos; and X_2 = indicator for a history of cigarette smoking. Note that the interaction effect associated with individuals who both smoked and were exposed to asbestos (X_1X_2) is almost four times larger than the next net largest coefficient. The much increased risk of death for people who fall into this category has significant implications for health education.

It is a safe bet that researchers and evaluators in the area of health policy face a comparable situation. In general, as the number of determinants and the range over which they vary increases, interaction effects also increase. A drug that exhibits no side-effects in a group of 15-21-year-old males may be found to cause numerous side-effects in the general population where the range of variation in blood pressure, circulatory problems, body weight, and kidney condition is much greater. HSAs and the environments in which they operate differ enormously on a large number of dimensions, and the number and magnitude of these differences make complex interaction effects highly probable. To further complicate matters, the impact of some determinants can be expected to interact with time itself as a result of learning behavior and adaptation. Because the enabling legislation permits planning agencies considerable choice in how, why, and when decisions are made, there is plenty of room for learning and adaptation to take place.

As a result, most variables in which researchers and policymakers are interested are likely to have a complex, contingent effect that cannot be usefully summarized with an elegant *ceteris paribus* statement or single regression coefficient. Neither the goals of HSA board members nor the activity of hospital associations and other interest groups has a simple impact on capital spending, hospital costs per day, or growth of HMO market share. That impact almost certainly depends on numerous other factors, ranging from the inflation rate to the qualification and experience of HSA staff--factors that can be expected to vary from place to place and over time.

Evidence of important interaction effects among key variables is slowly beginning to accumulate. A recent example is the Policy Analysis, Inc., *et al.* (1980) analysis of interstate variation in the certificate-of-need program. In chapter 2, considerable emphasis is placed on the finding that both "program will" (a commitment to the constraint of industry growth) and "program mandate" (scope

of coverage, absence of loopholes, etc.) function as necessary but not sufficient conditions for CON success. This
is equivalent to saying that the impact of variables in
either category depends on the values of variables in
the other category, i.e., that interaction exists between
the dimensions. Presumably, and it is certainly intuitively reasonable, the impact of HSA board member goals depends critically on the scope of the legal mandate that
enables them to pursue those goals. By the same reasoning,
the impact of legal provisions depends on the goals of
board members and the intensity of their commitment.

Once one begins thinking about the diverse components
of "program will" and "mandate" and the multitude of possible interaction effects among them, the complexity of
summarizing the impact of a given variable becomes evident.
It poses no great problem to include a simple multiplicative term to suggest that the impact of strength of the
CON law on capital expenditures will vary depending on
the number of applications submitted. Statistically and
conceptually this is easy to manage. Neither, however,
is true when the effect of CON law strength also inter-
acts with board priorities, staff expertise, the time-
lapsed since adoption, average age of capital assets,
inflation rate, and seven other variables--each of which
interact with each other. Under such conditions, inferences about an individual case from simplistically
modeled aggregate results become extremely hazardous and
the findings of any individual study (e.g., a case study
of CON in New Jersey) are inevitably idiosyncratic.

Interaction also places heavy demands on sample size.
If the sample size is small and the number of variables
large, interactive relationships are unlikely to be detected much less modeled correctly. When there is a high
a priori expectation that most variables will have a
contingent impact, research with a small sample may not
even be worth conducting. A related point is that special
care must be taken to maximize the variation on the independent variables. Any nonlinear relationship can
appear linear over a compact enough set of values. Obviously, if increased staff expertise leads to more
restrictive CON decisions only in HSAs with cost conscious
boards, an adequate number of such HSAs must be present
in the sample for this interaction to be detected.

Finally, when interaction is probable, it is very easy
to underestimate the importance of a particular variable
if that judgment is based solely on its linear coefficient.

Although the bivariate relationship between it and the dependent variable may be small or nonexistent, it may have an important interactive impact that would be lost if the variable were dismissed at an early stage of the exploratory analysis. For example, the degree to which states centralize the functions of health planning, certificate-of-need review, and rate-setting may, in and of itself, have little or no relationship with capital spending. Nonetheless, it is possible that it might have an important impact on the opportunity and ability of a governor to exert an influence.

PART 2: RESEARCH AND EVALUATION STRATEGIES

There is no simple research strategy that will magically accomplish the twin tasks of accurately assessing system performance and developing an effective technology of health planning and regulation, but the nature of the problems just described does suggest certain prescriptions about how evaluation, research, and analysis should proceed.

Prescription 1: Interpret Research Findings Cautiously

A central theme of the preceding section is that considerable caution must be exercised when evaluating research on the effects and effectiveness of the health planning system. This applies both to broad generalizations about what the system as a whole has accomplished and to judgments about the impact of any single component. Aggregate impact is difficult to assess partly because the mandate provided HSAs and SHPDAs encompasses aspects of service delivery that are hard to measure (e.g., access and quality) and partly because our ability to distinguish what occurred from what "would have" occurred without the law is less than is generally acknowledged. Restricting the scope of evaluation to certain costs of care and capital spending indicators solves the measurement problem but that of generating a reliable "counterfactual" remains. The accurate estimation of what would have happened without P.L. 93-641 requires models that can accurately forecast costs and capital spending, and these have yet to be developed.

Identifying the key determinants of outcome variation and estimating their individual effects are even more problematic. A disconcerting proportion of potentially important determinants (e.g., SHPDA-SHCC-HSA-PSRO relations, HSA goals) are difficult to access and quantify. Furthermore, multicollinearity arising from a large number of determinants and complex interaction effects can combine to cause serious errors in model specification and parameter estimates. The significance level attributed to a coefficient can greatly underestimate the uncertainty with which it should be viewed, and policy inferences about the effect of manipulating a particular factor are extremely risky. If research results appear to suggest that a policy change is in order, it should be implemented on a limited, trial basis and carefully monitored. It simply makes no sense to advocate wholesale reforms on the basis of a model estimated from nonexperimental data that can explain a mere 20 percent of the variance in a service delivery or outcome measure.

Prescription 2: Continue to Develop a Wide Range of Performance Measures That Encompass Service Delivery Outputs and Health Status Outcomes, but Take Care Not to Neglect the Decision-Making Process

A necessary prelude to accurately assessing the impact of health planning and acquiring the knowledge to make it more effective is the maintenance of trustworthy, quantitative performance measures. The systematic data collection and reporting requirements necessary to support this activity can play an important positive role in structuring the agenda of planning agencies and in quality control. Despite the occasional protestations of busy HSA staff, there is a substantial overlap between the data that are likely to be requested from state and federal agencies and those needed to engage in effective planning. Reporting requirements help ensure that each area of responsibility--cost control, access to care, etc.--will be accorded at least some minimal attention by HSAs and provide the evidence necessary for legislators and consumers to judge program results.

Serious attempts are now being completed in a number of quarters to construct quantitative performance measures that deal with the more elusive aspects of quality of care, access, and technology coordination and utilization. These are to be applauded not only because they play a central role in the basic charge given agencies by the 1974 act but because they are the areas where the limited regulatory authority granted planning agencies is most likely to bring positive results. The power of capital expenditure review to directly influence the major sources of cost increases is considerably less than their ability to affect access or technology coordination. One of the paradoxes of program evaluation in this area has been the minimal overlap between characteristics of the health care system for which high quality quantitative data are available and those characteristics which are likely to be affected by health planning.

This current emphasis on developing "hard" measures of planning effectiveness is a predictable (and overdue) response to the political pressure created by critics and competing expenditure categories. It is also a consequence of an increasingly sophisticated awareness of the limitations of information about process and compliance standards as a basis for allocating scarce economic resources. The ultimate justification for any health care policy decision is the anticipated impact on health status outcomes, and to ignore them is to risk the possibility of being interminably wrong-headed. As we have seen, however, there can be substantial inference problems in using outcome measures as the sole basis for evaluating the effectiveness of planning agencies. Outcome measures can be so influenced by statistically uncontrollable extraneous factors and/or be so difficult to measure that effectiveness inferences based on them can be inferior to those generated by process data.

Suppose that we are interested in evaluating the progress that a given HSA has made in ensuring equal access to medical care for certain subgroups of the population. One way to do this would be to chart changes in morbidity and mortality rates for these groups and then compare them with those of the general population. Another would be to study utilization rates. A third would be to gather data on the decisions made by the HSA and the nature of the evidence or arguments that were presented in support of those decisions. The first approach deals directly with outcomes but the amount of confidence with which we can attribute any changes to interventions on the part of the HSA is going to be small. Any number of factors could have been responsible for whatever changes take place and health status outcomes are often unresponsive in the short run to any type of intervention. Utilization measures generally have less lag time associated with them, but the problem of linking access change directly to HSA activity is not substantially reduced. Only the study of HSA decision-making will provide dependable evidence of HSA interest in unequal access and both the character and intensity of their efforts to ameliorate the problem. It would be silly to argue that the third strategy should be pursued to the exclusion of the other two since it tells us nothing about impact. However, it provides the kind of critical collaborative evidence necessary to establish linkages between planning and outcomes. Without such evidence it may be possible to evaluate the performance of a health service *area* but *not* that of a health system *agency*.

Reference to outcome measures alone will never enable us to learn what HSA actions are the most effective or why one HSA succeeds and another fails. To answer these questions it is necessary to probe inside the "black box" of planning agency decision processes in much the same way that private firms and other regulatory agencies are studied. Analytical case studies of HSA decision-making in the tradition of Altman (1978) and Bauer (1978), which attempt to capture the political and bureaucratic dynamics of health planning are an important beginning. However, systematic modeling of HSA decision-making along the lines begun by Luft and Frisvold (1979) has received far too little attention.

Prescription 3: Employ Longitudinal Data

We have just seen how an overly narrow perspective about which variables should be measured can restrict the quality of inferences that can be drawn. The same is true for the period of time covered by the research. One source of error lies in expecting too much too soon. As Roucheleau (1980:605) has recently argued, complex intergovernmental programs require an extended developmental period. Time is necessary to cultivate the networks of formal and informal relations that are needed to make them effective. Moreover, many of the policy choices that are made can be expected to have a delayed or cumulative effect that cannot be detected in the short run. For example, the impact of a consumer education program might only be evident after several years. Restricting the time period that is analyzed also makes it impossible to chart adaptive behavior. This is particularly troublesome because we have every reason to expect that learning behavior and adaptation are critical elements in any regulatory environment. In addition, from a purely methodological standpoint, observations over several years are often necessary to increase the N to a point where interactive relationships can be detected.

It is even possible that the contexts in which planning agencies operate and the nature of the agencies themselves differ along so many dimensions that no single model can accurately characterize or predict their behavior. Aggregate data analysis and comparative studies have their limitations. Trying to make sense out of a data set that contains towns with a population of 500, as well as Chicago and Tokyo, can be a fruitless endeavor, and there is no guarantee that HSAs or SHPDAs represent a more homogeneous population. The analyst who proceeds with a comparative study of HSAs may face the unpleasant task of choosing between a parsimonious and interpretable model that is capable of explaining only a small amount of variance and contains coefficients with large standard errors and a specification in which the variables and their interactions are too numerous to estimate with the amount of data available. In this situation, it is advisable to examine the units of analysis individually over time, especially from the perspective of estimating program impact. This is true because a number of dimensions that might be critical in explaining performance variation across HSAs or states (e.g., CON provisions, interest group strength) will be effectively held constant in the individual case and can be ignored. The result is a simpler model that is limited with respect to the generalizations that can be drawn but more useful.

Prescription 4: Acknowledge the High Probability of Substantial Interaction Among Variables and Employ Appropriate Data Analysis Techniques

The relative absence of theoretical direction in this area places a heavy responsibility on the techniques of exploratory analysis and the analyst. A substantial part of this responsibility lies in acknowledging the likelihood of complex interaction effects and searching for them. Ideally, the detection of interaction is relatively straightforward. The analyst can proceed by creating bivariate multiplicative terms and then checking for

significance. Such simple multiplicative terms may be
a long way from a correct specification of the interaction
that is actually taking place, but it is a useful place
to begin. The expectation is that the presence of interaction will be detected through this procedure and that
a more sophisticated statistical analysis--looking at
higher orders of interaction with alternative functional
forms--can then proceed. Naturally, if the number of
variables in the data set is large, even the number of
bivariate combinations can be imposing enough to warrant
the use of a simple computer program to assist in the
search.

Detecting interaction becomes more challenging when
it involves a variable that has been measured and one or
more that have been omitted from the analysis. Unquestionably, the instability of coefficients over time and cases
is the most prominent indicator of interaction with an
omitted variable(s). Epidemiologists studying cancer,
for example, suspect that a carcinogen has an interactive
impact if the incidence of cancer per unit of exposure
varies over time or increases with the age of the sample.
In both cases the tentative presumption is that the changes
in the effect of the carcinogen are brought about by
variation in exposure to background factors. The same
logic is relevant to research on health planning. If the
coefficient reflecting the impact of HSA priorities changes
over time or from one state to another, suspect interaction
and search for the variables involved.[2] While it is clear
that the nature of the interaction and the predictions that
it would lead to are ultimately inaccessible without direct
measurement of the relevant variable, any indication of
its existence can be helpful. At best this will inspire
the search for a better understanding of the behavior/
phenomenon in question; at worst it will prepare the
decision-maker for a rash of unintended consequences.

The simple step of checking for interactions by including power and product terms in a regression could, if
widely practiced, make the problems of interaction and
nonlinearity much more visible. There are, however,
definite limitations to the technique. In the first place,
interaction is often accompanied by residual nonnormality,
which can result in difficult inferential problems even
if sufficient interaction terms are included to follow the
curvature. Secondly, if the number of variables in a
problem grows to any size at all, the number of interactive
terms needed becomes unwieldy. A model with six basic

variables and all possible interaction terms up to the sixth-order interaction would require estimating nearly 1,000 coefficients.

Possible aid in dealing with these problems lies in the use of variable transformations. When carefully chosen, these transformations can simultaneously reduce heteroscedacticity, nonnormal error distributions, and the degree of interaction. If in the lung cancer death rate example given earlier, the logarithm of each variable is used in place of the raw scores the regression becomes

$$\ln(\hat{Y}) = 2.42 + 1.65\ln X_1 + 2.39\ln X_2 = 0.06(\ln X_1)(\ln X_2).$$

and the previously huge interaction is virtually elim-inated.[3]

While the application of transformations should reduce interaction effects, it would be overly optimistic to believe that they will invariably bring them under control. There are going to be times when the level of interaction is so great that accurate estimation or coherent inter-pretation will be impossible. When this situation arises, an attempt may be made to simplify the analysis problem by reducing the number of variables in the model or by searching for new variables used that do not interact as heavily. Frequently, both strategies are pursued simul-taneously by employing a dimensionality reducing technique such as factor analysis, principal components analysis, or multidimensional scaling. Unfortunately, these methods are usable only with linear data and tend to obscure rather than reveal important interactions.

Whatever method is used to select and estimate the model, the presence of a large number of variables and potential interactions can result in models containing terms that correspond to no real effect. The most reliable answer to this problem is the use of data splitting methods, of which the simplest is to select and estimate the model using half of the data and then test it on the other half. This helps prevent an overly optimistic assessment of the explanatory power of a model that has been chosen for the best fit to the data at hand.

Prescription 5: Utilize Experimental Designs to Evaluate Policy Alternatives Whenever Possible

The inference problems that have been described in the preceding pages could be dramatically reduced if experimenta

designs were more widely employed. There is no doubt
that a properly designed experiment yields both more and
better-quality information than an observational study.
Although there are areas where a proper design would be
politically unfeasible, unethical, or too costly, there
are fewer than is frequently assumed.

The only way to be sure which of two policy alternatives is superior is to try them both out under similar
conditions. If one is interested in learning whether
capital expenditure caps are more effective in reducing
costs than CONs, comparing the respective performances
of states or HSAs that have implemented one or the other
could be a waste of time. Any number of secular trends
can masquerade as program effects and the depth of our
ignorance about what is really going on combined with
the complexities involved make it much more difficult
than usual to statistically control for their influence.
Only by systematically choosing some units to implement
the spending caps while others use CONs and then simultaneously observing the outcomes can a valid comparison
be made.

The primary basis for choosing the treatment and
control groups for policy experiments, as in clinical
experiments, should be randomization. Experience has
shown that it is risky to assign groups by any other
means, including judgmental balancing. This is especially
true in areas such as health care policy, where there are
so many possible sources of confounding effects. When
randomization is used, consideration should be given to
the use of nonparametric randomization tests that are
exactly valid. Most of the time, however, normal theory
methods provide an adequate approximation to the randomization tests.

For those who still think of experimental design exclusively in terms of varying a single factor while
holding all others fixed, the suggestion that it should
be more widely employed may seem prohibitively inefficient.
We are, after all, often interested in learning about the
impact of more than one policy alternative, as well as
detecting interaction effects. Yet as R. A. Fisher first
demonstrated almost 40 years ago, testing several variables
simultaneously greatly increases the efficiency of the
design and can also be used to detect interaction. Suppose, for example, that it is felt that a cap on building
expenditures is often an ineffective cost reduction tactic
because the same funds are simply channeled toward the

purchase of new equipment. This is equivalent to sus-
pecting a serious interaction between plant expenditure
caps and equipment expenditure caps. It is equally plausible that the level of HSA/SHPDA staff expertise and other
environmental conditions may interact with both. For-
tunately, all of these interactions can be revealed by a
thoughtfully constructed factorial or fractional factorial
experimental design. As increasing attention shifts to
reforming the present system of health planning and
regulation the opportunity and need for policy experiments
will also increase. Reforms such as capital and operating
cost caps, investment subsidies, and reimbursement controls
should be evaluated at the earliest opportunity using
sophisticated experimental designs.

CONCLUSION

The future of health planning is inextricably bound to
policy research and evaluation. If adequate funding and
organizational support for these activities is not forthcoming, the results are all too predictable. Program
evaluation will consist of nothing more than "scorecard"
recordings of cost increases, capital expenditures, the
percentage of CON applications approved, and the degree
to which HSAs and SHPDAs are in compliance with the structural and procedural requirements of the Health Planning
Act and its amendments. The politically delicate and
quantitatively elusive areas of responsibility such as
quality of care will be effectively ignored despite the
fact that they may be more directly influenced by HSA
decisions than can cost. Because the major focus will
be on charting outcomes rather than on acquiring a better
understanding of the relative impact of alternative policy
strategies, structural configurations, and incentive
arrangements, next to nothing will be learned about why
the system is working as well or poorly as it is or how
it might be improved.

This failure to improve the knowledge base and technology of planning will, in turn, ensure that policy debates continue to be dominated by theoretical speculations
about the probable role of various incentives for utility
maximizing consumers and institutions. Policymakers will
be left to cope as best they can with arguments that assure
them that only HMOs can provide adequate incentives for
physicians to use hospitals less and aggressively promote
health maintenance or, conversely, that the same incentives

might discourage their keeping a patient alive who
requires long-term treatment.

In the midst of uncertainty about quality-access-
cost trade-offs and in the absence of statistically
defensible review standards, health planning and regulation
will flounder. Providers will attack formal HSA decision
criteria as arbitrary and insensitive to important contextual considerations. State and federal agencies will
criticize the absence of such criteria as demonstrating
a lack of commitment to planning. The inconsistent and
tentative HSA behavior that will almost inevitably result from the confluence of these forces will be interpreted by outside observers as indicative of the fundamentally "political" behavior of HSA boards--even when
it might better be described as the by-product of a profound uncertainty about what to do and how to do it.
Politics has always had a way of filling analytic vacuums
for both decision-makers and social scientists.

What is ironic in view of their central role in the
health planning system is that HSA/SHPDA behavior will
have relatively little influence on whether the above
scenario comes true or not. Whatever their merits as
instruments through which to express community values,
from a cognitive and information processing perspective
they are neither particularly efficient nor effective.
With few exceptions, they do not possess the staffs or
resources necessary to competently assess decision alternatives or evaluate their subsequent impact. If a well-
developed technology of planning and regulation existed
or if the issues they faced were less complex, things might
be different--but neither is the case.

There are organizational imperatives associated with
knowledge development and evaluation that are no less
powerful than those arising from economic constraints and
political interests. If ignored, they exact the same high
cost. In this case it is absolutely essential that leadership and resources come from outside. Some external agency
must make decisions about what data will be collected
and maintained, ensure that they are properly analyzed,
and make formal provision for their dissemination. I am
not describing here the traditionally passive function of
those state and federal agencies that make data available
upon demand and issue periodic reports that summarize
emerging trends.[4] Nor am I describing what is usually
thought of as quality control. What is at issue here is
the generation of detailed analyses of the major policy

options facing planning agencies and exhaustive evaluations
of their decisions and programs.

How the burden of providing these services should be
divided between federal and state agencies is too complex
a question to be resolved here. DHHS and its Bureau of
Health Planning house greater expertise than most state
agencies and have long assumed a leadership role in this
area. Documents such as their *Guidelines of the Acquisition and Use of Data under Public Law 93-641* have already
provided local planning agencies with much needed direction. On the other hand, state officials are often in the
best position to appreciate critical contextual variations,
frequently enjoy more operational flexibility than their
federal counterparts, and face a more manageable analytic
task since they deal with many fewer HSAs and only one
SHPDA. Two things are certain, however. Some agency or
combination of agencies must assume the responsibilities
described in the preceding paragraph if the health planning system is to function properly and much higher levels
of funding will be required to support their efforts.

NOTES

1. The sources of exogenous shocks range from changes
in unemployment and inflation to unilateral decisions made
by insurers and often governmental agencies.

2. If one or more other interacting independent variables is missing, it is obviously impossible to stratify a
cross-sectional data set in such a way as to reveal coefficient instability. However, even under these conditions it is still possible to identify potentially significant interaction effects by searching for heteroscedacticity or inequality of error variance (see Downs and Rocke,
1979).

3. There are a number of ways to select the most appropriate transformation. Probably the simplest and most
common tactic is to choose the logarithm or square root
based on *a priori* considerations. Thus an economist who
assumes that production Y is related to labor X_1 and
capital X_2 by

$$Y = b_0 X_1^{b_1} X_2^{b_2}$$

may choose to take logarithms before analyzing the data
and fit

$$\log Y = b_0 + b_1 \log X_1 + b_2 \log X_2.$$

Another form of *a priori* choice of transportation involves a set of rules used by data analysts called "first aid for data" (Mosteller and Tukey, 1977). In brief, and slightly simplified, the rules call for logarithms with measured data, square roots for counted data, and logits for proportions. Although rules like these or guidance from prespecified models may be helpful, ultimately a transformation must be justifiable from the data. It would be foolish to accept an *a priori* transformation (or an *a priori* lack of transformation) without checking the adequacy of the choice.

Purely data-based transformations can be accomplished in several ways. Typically the choice is between various power transformations X^λ or $\log X$ (which corresponds to $\lambda = 0$) and the usual procedure is to choose that which maximizes normality (Box and Cox, 1964) or symmetry (Tukey, 1977). Transformations are done separately for each independent and the dependent variable. The logic behind this procedure is that variables measured on the "wrong" scale lead to nonlinearity, interaction, heteroscedactivity, and nonnormality and that a transformation chosen to eliminate nonnormality can also do a good job of reducing the others. It is also possible to base the choice of transformation directly on reduction of nonlinearity. A rather simple way to do this is to transform the dependent variable guided by symmetry or homoscedasticity and then to choose the transformation of each independent variable by trial and error if necessary, so as to maximize the bivariate r^2. Even more effective might be to estimate the transformations simultaneously with the coefficients by nonlinear least-squares.

4. I am also proposing something that goes beyond section 1501 of P.L. 96-79, which requires DHHS to "collect data to determine whether the health care delivery systems meet or are changing to meet the goals included in health systems plans."

REFERENCES AND BIBLIOGRAPHY

Aday, Lu Ann (1980). "Access to Medical Care in the United States: Equitable for Whom?" Paper delivered at the Conference on National Health Policy, Stanford, Calif.
Altman, Drew (1978). "The Politics of Health Care Regulation: The Case of the National Health Planning and

112

Resources Development Act." *Journal of Health Politics, Policy and Law* 2(Winter):560-580.

Bauer, Katherine G. (1978). *Cost Containment Under P.L. 93-641.* Boston: Harvard University Center for Community Health and Medical Care Report Series R58-8.

Berry, Ralph E., Jr. (1978). "Research Needs for Future Policy" in *Hospital Cost Containment.* M. Zubkoft, I. Raskin, and R. S. Hanft, eds. New York: Prodist.

Bicknell, William, and Diana Chapman Walsh (1975). "Certificate of Need: The Massachusetts Experience." *New England Journal of Medicine* 292:20, 1054-1061.

Box, George E. P., and D. R. Cox (1964). "An Analysis of Transformation." *Journal of the Royal Statistical Society* B26:211-252.

Bureau of Health Planning (1978). *Guidelines for the Acquisition and Use of Data Under P.L. 93-641.* Washington, D.C.: DHEW Publication No. 78-14013.

Bureau of Health Planning (1980). *Toward a Better Health System: Annual Report Fiscal 1979.* Washington, D.C.: U.S. Department of Health and Human Services.

Cain, Harry P., and Helen Darling (1979). "Health in the United States: Where We Stand Today." *Health Policy and Education* 1:5-25.

Cronbach, Lee J. (1976). "Beyond the Two Disciplines of Scientific Psychology." *American Psychologist* 30:2, 116-121.

Downs, George W., and David M. Rocke (1979). "Interpreting Heteroscedasticity." *American Journal of Political Science* 23:4, 816-829.

Hammond, E. Cuyler (1979). "Partitioning the Blame; Problems of Interactions." Address given at the Annual Meeting of the American Statistical Association, Washington, D.C.

Levin, Arthur (ed.) (1980). *Regulating Health Care.* New York: Academy of Political Science.

Luft, Harold S., and Gary A. Frisvold (1979). "Decision Making in Regional Health Planning Agencies." *Journal of Health Politics, Policy and Law* 2:250-272.

McAuliffe, William E. (1979). "Measuring the Quality of Medical Care: Process Versus Outcome." *Milbank Memorial Fund Quarterly/Health and Society* 57:1, 118-152.

Mosteller, Frederick, and John W. Tukey (1977). *Data Analysis.* Reading, Mass.: Addison-Wesley.

Newhouse, T. P. (1974). "A Design for a Health Insurance Experiment." *Inquiry* 11:5-27.

Policy Analysis, Inc. and Urban Systems Research & Engineering, Inc. *Evaluation of the Effects of Certificate of Need Programs*, HRA #230-7F-0165, Washington, D.C., Department of Health and Human Services, August 1980.

Rocheleau, Bruce (1980). "How Do We Measure the Impact of Intergovernmental Programs? Some Problems and Examples from the Health Area." *Journal of Health Politics, Policy and Law* 4:4, 605-619.

Russell, Louise B. (1979). *Technology in Hospitals*. Washington, D.C.: Brookings.

Salkever, David S., and Thomas W. Bice (1979). *Hospital Certificate of Need Controls*. Washington, D.C.: American Enterprise Institute.

Schneider, Don (1980). "Economic Impact and Project Selection Methodology for Certificate of Need." Final report submitted to New York State Health Planning Commission.

Schultze, Charles L. (1968). *The Politics and Economics of Public Spending*. Washington, D.C.: Brookings.

Schweitzer, Stuart (1978). "Health Care Cost-Containment Programs: An International Perspective." In *Hospital Cost Containment*. M. Zubkoff, I. Raskin, and R. S. Hanft, eds. New York: Prodist.

Sterman, Arnold B., and Herbert H. Schaumberg (1980). "The Role of the Cranial CT Scan in Municipal Hospitals." *American Journal of Public Health* 70:3, 268-270.

Sweetland, Margaret, Drew Altman, and Eugene W. Matter (1978). *Institutional Responses to Evolving Health Planning and Regulatory Programs*. Boston: Harvard Center for Community Health and Medical Care Report Series R58-7.

Tukey, John W. (1977). *Exploratory Data Analysis*. Reading, Mass.: Addison-Wesley.

NATIONAL/STATE/LOCAL
RELATIONSHIPS IN HEALTH PLANNING:
INTEREST GROUP REACTION
AND LOBBYING*

G. Gregory Raab

*Understanding the weaknesses, strengths, and structural
components of health planning in the United States today
is considerably aided by an understanding of the controversies, interest group positions, and negotiations that
occurred before the National Health Planning and Resources
Development Act was passed and regulations issued. In
this paper Raab traces the history of the act and regulations, describing the involvement of congressional and
other actors in the development process. The outcome
of that process is the intricate balance of national,
state, and local planning relationships that exists today.*

The controversies that accompanied the legislative drafting and the administrative implementation of the National
Health Planning and Resources Development Act (Public
Law 93-641) have tended to center on two issues. The
first concerns the planning law's regulatory (and other
review) provisions that expand the government's control
over the traditionally private health care system. These
provisions require the administration of satisfactory
certificate-of-need programs in each state, the review of
a wide range of federal health funds by local planning
agencies, the periodic review of existing health services
and facilities in order to determine their appropriateness,

---

*The views herein are those of the author and are not
necessarily those of the Health Care Financing Administration or the U.S. Department of Health and Human Services.

114

and national support for prospective rate-setting experiments in a number of states. These review functions, in combination with the requirement in Public Law 93-641 that each planning agency develop and carry out specific health plans, signaled a distinct change in direction for the federal government. They marked the end of the congressional prohibition against interference with the private practice of medicine that had characterized the earlier comprehensive health planning program, and they portended even more regulation for the future.

Quite naturally, these provisions attracted a great deal of medical interest group attention and lobbying as they were considered by the Congress and implemented by HEW. Both congressional sponsors of increased health regulation and federal administrators expected this opposition, considered it legitimate, and dealt pragmatically in negotiating with medical interest groups. However, a second issue raised by the new planning law provoked controversies of equal importance to those generated by the regulatory provisions of Public Law 93-641, and it mobilized interest groups with little experience in lobbying national health policymakers.

This second issue concerns the organizational ground rules for the new health planning effort. The structural provisions of Public Law 93-641 modified intergovernmental relationships that delegated substantial responsibility for administering domestic policies to state and local elected officials. This delegation began in the last years of the Johnson administration and was formalized in the new federalism principles advocated by the Nixon administration. The health planning law's bias toward special-purpose substate planning agencies organized on a private nonprofit (instead of a public) basis and the detailed conditions and requirements placed on state officials in the new health planning/regulation system were not consistent with the new federalism, and these structural provisions led state and local elected officials (and their Washington representatives) to enter the health policy-making process. This paper outlines the basis for state and local governmental lobbying with respect to the planning structure mandated by Public Law 93-641, it indicates the degree to which congressional sponsors and federal administrators of the new planning law considered its regulatory goals to be dependent upon new national, state, and local governmental relationships, and it presents an overview of the major disputes that occurred between HEW administrators of the planning program and state and local elected officials.

THE NATIONAL HEALTH PLANNING LAW

Congressman William R. Roy, a member of the Subcommittee on Health and the Environment of the House Interstate and Foreign Commerce Committee, summarized the mood of the Congress toward health planning in early 1974, when he said: "Health planning without government regulation to enforce it just doesn't work."[1] This congressional inclination to remedy what had been identified as one of the most serious drawbacks of comprehensive health planning constituted a major shift in policy for the Congress, and it drew the attention of lobbyists who had previously paid little attention to the subject of health planning. This attention grew more intense as it became apparent that the policy decisions made in drafting the new health planning statute would be central to any future program of national health insurance.[2] A sound health planning effort was considered to be a necessary first step for national health insurance, and planning supporters hoped to head off an escalation in costs similar to that which had followed enactment of the Medicare and Medicaid legislation. Although there was substantial consensus on this point within both subcommittees having jurisdiction over the health planning program and the administration, there were major differences of opinion expressed on the extent of health regulation necessary to control health costs (and to promote improvements in the access to and quality of health care), as well as the organizational characteristics of the planning agencies that would administer it. These differences of opinion, resolved in the statutory provisions of Public Law 93-641, continued as the national health planning law was implemented.

BACKGROUND

Both the substantive goals of the new health planning law and the structural provisions to meet these goals were developed and made explicit as a direct result of federal experience gained from administering the prior comprehensive health planning program authorized by Public Law 89-749. The most obvious constraint of Public Law 89-749 was its proscription against interference with the private

practice of medicine,[3] and each of the various bills given
serious consideration by Congress as a replacement for
the comprehensive health planning program proposed to
add significant regulatory authority. However, there
were other factors that guided the Congress as it considered the particulars of a new health planning law.
These factors included: a desire to secure tangible program results; a skepticism regarding the abilities of
existing national, state, and local agencies and organizations that had been entrusted with the voluntary comprehensive health planning effort; an emphasis on a technocratic and rational health planning process (and a con-
comitant distrust of politics and politicians who, it was
feared, would disregard or overturn planning agency determinations); and a commitment to the principle that
health planning should attract the interest and involvement
of community leaders in order to ensure its relevance and
legitimacy.[4]

As a result, the planning bills that were drafted and
considered by the House and Senate health subcommittees
were highly specific, detailed, and prescriptive.[5] While
they provided greater national funding and direction to
state and substate health planning efforts, they also
restricted the discretion customarily granted HEW in administering health programs. Congressional interests
understood that HEW had provided little direction or technical assistance to comprehensive health planning agencies
and that a more active national presence would be required
if the substantive goals of any new health planning legislation were to be achieved. Further, the bills were
written with a specificity more characteristic of administrative regulations than authorizing legislation in order
to guarantee the timely implementation of the new planning
program. Health subcommittee staff wanted to avoid the
delays inherent in HEW's rulemaking process by providing
in statute most of the details necessary to secure prompt
administrative action in establishing the new health planning structure.[6]

Similarly, the bills attempted to isolate the health
planning process at the state and local levels from any
possible political interference. For example, H.R. 12053,
the bill introduced by Paul G. Rogers, chairman of the
Interstate and Foreign Commerce Committee's Health Subcommittee, and co-sponsored by Health Subcommittee members
William R. Roy and James F. Hastings, required state-level
health planning to be conducted by specially established,
consumer-dominated commissions empowered with broad

regulatory authority. The commissions were to carry out
their activities according to a detailed "administrative
program" approved by the secretary of HEW; failure to
perform these functions satisfactorily after 4 years
would result in the HEW secretary performing them in place
of the state. At the local level, this bill required
health planning agencies to be organized as special-
purpose, private nonprofit corporations composed of consumers, providers, and public elected officials, each
grouping receiving one-third representation on the planning agency's governing board. The bill also gave
specific direction with respect to both the organization
and staffing of these agencies and their plan-development
and plan-implementation activities.

Congressional interest in the administrative structuring
of health programs was a recent development. Until the
late 1960s, national policymakers were preoccupied with
the substantive goals of health policy (i.e., targeting
funds to defined groups through categorical health programs,
providing support for medical research, and making available financial assistance for hospital construction); they
usually neglected the way in which federal health programs
were administered. They considered public sector relationships with private medical interests to be of paramount
concern as they developed health policy, and they assumed
that state and local elected officials could be counted
on to provide the health services or to administer the
controls on the health system that were increasingly required by federal statutes. However, as a result of the
conflicts and disruptions associated with implementing
Great Society programs in the mid 1960s, as well as the
poor record set by state and local officials in administering the 1966 comprehensive health planning law, national
policymakers came to recognize the degree to which federal
grant programs were dependent upon subnational officials
for their success in meeting national objectives. The
structural provisions of the 1974 health planning law
were a deliberate attempt by national officials to reduce
this dependency through organizational requirements that
either bypassed or limited the discretion of elected
officials at the state and local levels. The new planning
law called for more centralized intergovernmental relationships in order to ensure that its regulatory (and other
review) provisions would be successful in controlling
the escalating costs of health care.

Planning Structure

As enacted, Public Law 93-641 departed from earlier planning laws by prescribing in detail the organizational
arrangement through which planning agencies would implement their new regulatory tools. Because the broad
statutory mandate given the comprehensive health planning
program too often had resulted in only sporadic HEW
direction and only scattered success for state and substate regional planning agencies, Congress chose to give
explicit statutory direction to the national, state, and
local health planning effort. Where the earlier voluntary
planning program had been consistent with a governmental
movement in the late 1960s to decentralize health decision-
making, the new planning law was characterized by greater
centralization and tighter federal surveillance and
standard-setting.[7] Briefly, HEW was to provide national
direction and standards, financial support, and technical
assistance to state and local health planning agencies;
state agencies were responsible for the distinctly governmental function of health regulation; and substate agencies
were to bring together representatives of the pluralistic
(and essentially private) health system by planning for
the health needs of their geographic areas and by providing state and national decision-makers with advice on
how to exercise their regulatory controls on the health
sector. At the state level, private advisory councils,
instead of state officials, were to integrate local plans
for the health system and to approve the state's health
plan.

State and local elected officials and their Washington
representatives were preoccupied with Richard Nixon's Watergate crisis during 1973 and 1974, when the new planning
bill was being developed; they gave health planning little
chance of passage in the new federalism era of block grants
and special revenue sharing. However, as the new planning
law took shape in the Congress, state and local governmental
interests objected to the structure of health planning.
To these elected officials and the groups that represented
them, the health planning structure mandated by Public
Law 93-641 bypassed elected officials, undermined state
and local prerogatives, raised the specter of national
control over functions that had traditionally been reserved
for state and local governments, and permitted the dominance
of federal program specialists in HEW over state and local
governmental generalists.[8] The combination of health

planning and regulatory activities in the new planning
law raised issues centered on the allocation of power
among national, state, and local governments, and it
brought a new participant to the specialized discussions
and negotiations normally conducted among congressional
health subcommittee members and staff, HEW program
specialists, and medical interest groups. The involvement of state and local elected officials in health
planning brought to the fore basic questions with respect
to the operation of the federal system.

In particular, the state and local governmental lobby
sought increased discretion for state and local elected
officials in order to promote the public accountability
of the health planning program. Before the new planning
law was enacted, this group found particularly annoying
the provision in the leading House and Senate planning
bills, as well as the administration bill, requiring
local planning agencies to be organized on a private nonprofit basis. An editorial in *County News,* a weekly
publication of the National Association of Counties (NACo),
summarized the position of state and local elected officials toward this requirement:

> . . . federally mandated programs started without
> the support of local elected officials are bound
> to fail. Most state and Federal health services
> are delivered at the county level. It follows
> that local involvement will determine a program's
> success or failure. Citizens do not care who sup-
> ports the service. They just demand action from
> their local elected officials if that service is
> inadequate or nonexistent. . . .
> We fail to see how this proposal jibes with New
> Federalism. Turning over power to health providers
> not only runs counter to recent enactments as
> general revenue sharing, law enforcement, manpower,
> transportation and community development reform,
> but violates a cornerstone of American political
> philosophy: that power and accountability be kept
> as close to home as possible.[9]

To federal program officials and to congressional
sponsors of the health planning legislation and their
staff, the view of federalism advanced by this lobby
represented a challenge to a nonpartisan and nonpolitical
health planning process. With respect to the private

nonprofit organizational status of substate planning
agencies, the report of the House Commerce Committee
accompanying its version of the planning bill made
the following points: (1) the bulk of the comprehensive
health planning agencies authorized by Public Law 89-749
were organized as private nonprofit entities and had
operated in this way for several years; (2) most expenditures in the health field came from private, not
public, sources, and it was reasonable for planning agencies to reflect this fact; and (3) the congressional
sponsors of health planning were aware of several instances
where the public governing board of local planning
agencies (such as councils of governments and regional
planning commissions) had reversed, for political reasons,
the recommendations of their health advisors.[10] The
state and local governmental lobby was, nevertheless,
successful in enlisting the support of Congressman Moss,
then chairman of the Oversight Subcommittee of the
House Commerce Committee; with Moss' backing the House
measure was amended to permit the designation of public
substate planning agencies. This lobby also succeeded in
convincing the Senate Health Subcommittee to include
public agencies as eligible applicants for substate planning grants.

State and local elected officials also opposed the
nature of the state-level health planning apparatus that
had been specified in the House Bill, H.R. 12053. Soon
after H.R. 12053 was introduced, Kevin McKenna, special
counsel to Rhode Island Governor Philip W. Noel, commented
that the House bill "completely bypasses the Governors"
by requiring that state-level health planning be performed
by independent commissions which "lack straight-line
accountability." He stated further that:

The commission form that they are developing is a
throwback to the days when commissions ran state
government. It usually means that the interest
groups predominate on those commissions and they
are not accountable to the elected representatives
of the people.

We're not opposed to the purposes of the bill,
but the administrative mechanisms that have been
proposed for implementing those purposes I'm afraid
could be counter-productive, so we will bring that
to the attention of the Senate and House subcommittees.[11]

The drafters of H.R. 12053 feared placing governors in a position to influence state health planning for the same reasons that they favored private nonprofit substate agencies--state governmental officials represented a political threat to professional health planning activities. However, House subcommittee staff reluctantly concluded that, despite the poor record of state government in managing health programs, the ambitious regulatory activities of H.R. 12053 would require state action in order to be implemented. As one staff person put it:

> We were not willing to create new government agencies at the local level and there are too many municipal governments anyway. We were not willing to concentrate all of this power in Washington. So what we were left with was the states.[12]

The mandated use of independent commissions in H.R. 12053 was an attempt to structure a special-purpose, professionally oriented agency at the state level that was at once capable of exercising state regulatory authority and independent of partisan influence. Senate health planning sponsors shared the House assessment of state governmental capabilities and attempted to draft a bill that would bypass the state altogether by placing health regulatory powers at either the national or substate regional levels.[13]

It should also be noted that HEW shared congressional concern that health planning be protected, to the extent practicable, from political influences. Consequently, the administration's planning bill required the designation of only private nonprofit agencies at the substate regional level. However, the administration favored a less directive approach toward the states. The administration's bill proposed to leave questions of state-level organization to the governors of the various states. The national health planning law, as enacted, relied on single-state agencies instead of independent commissions to perform state health planning and regulatory functions, and it permitted the delegation of specific responsibilities to other agencies of state government upon the request of the governor.

CHECKS AND BALANCES

Public Law 93-641 was the result of a deliberate choice by national health policymakers to promote intergovernmental

and public sector/private sector competition. A key
reason for the failure of the comprehensive health planning law had been the poor performance of HEW administrators and state governments, and the lack of involvement
of many community leaders (including local elected
officials) on planning agency governing boards had led to
that program's low visibility and, in many instances, to
its dominance by health care providers. The new law raised
the political importance of health planning by combining
planning and regulatory activities; in this way, it drew
the attention and the interest of public and private
actors to the structure of health planning. However,
the wording of the planning statute required that public
and private interests be mixed at the substate level,
permitting no one faction to achieve dominance on health
systems agency governing boards; similarly, prescribed
statutory roles for HEW, state governments, and local
health planning agencies, each influencing but not controlling its counterparts, kept any one actor from
directing (and possibly undermining) the planning/regula-
tion process. The emphasis on intergovernmental and
public/private conflict in the national health planning
law was an understandable by-product of the failures of
Public Law 89-749, and it was consciously intended by
supporters of a rational health planning process in the
Congress, in HEW, and at the local level who distrusted
the agents on whom the program must rely in order to
achieve substantive planning goals. Thus, although
Public Law 93-641 added significant regulatory and other
review responsibilities to health planning, the structural
dimension of planning remained a crucial concern of health
planning supporters--it was a guarantee that the strengthened program would achieve the desired results.[14]

Congress resolved in the statutory language of Public
Law 93-641 the dilemma of expanding the role of government
in health without establishing a national solution to the
particular problems associated with health care delivery
in each community. The national health planning law
built on existing intergovernmental and public sector/
private sector relationships in the health field, and it
transferred to new organizational forms and processes the
responsibility for managing the conflict associated with
expanded public control over a private industry. In its
reliance on state (rather than national) authority to
implement health planning decisions, and in its "gradual-
istic 'process' orientation and its pluralistic, multilevel

assignment of authority,"[15] Public Law 93-641 can even
be viewed as a rather conservative statute. The checks
and balances that were built into the new health planning
system presented opportunities for public and private
interests to achieve increased (or to maintain existing)
power in the health system, as well as the possibility
to suffer diminished influence and control over health
policy. Because the new health planning process threatened
the independence and perquisites that traditionally had
been enjoyed by health providers and state and local elected officials, the controversies concerning the operation of
the new health planning system, first raised before congressional health subcommittees, were transferred to HEW
as it developed regulations to provide the operational
ground rules for health planning. Two major issues addressed by HEW in regulation illustrated the new dimensions of the federal system in the mid-1970s. The first
issue dealt with the public accountability of health systems
agencies; the second concerned the administrative flexibility of each state to meet in its own way the substantive
goals set forth by the planning law.

Public Accountability

The first HEW regulations issued to implement Public
Law 93-641 governed the designation and funding of health
systems agencies (HSAs). Both congressional supporters
of health planning and HEW officials preferred the organization of local health planning agencies on a private
nonprofit basis, but, under intense pressure from state
and local officials, the planning law was written to
permit public regional planning bodies and single units
of general-purpose local government to be eligible for
HSA designation. However, several statutory and practical
barriers stood in the way of such designation,[16] and even
when public agencies were willing and able to compete for
and to secure designation as HSAs, the planning law diluted
their influence and control over the health planning ap-
paratus--it required a public agency to establish a separate
governing body for health planning with "exclusive authority"
to perform the agency's planning and review functions.[17]
The governing body for health planning was required to
meet the planning law's prescribed mix of consumers, providers, and public elected officials, and it was, to a
large degree, insulated from the public HSA's governing

board (or parent body), such as a county board of
supervisors or a regional council of governments. To
some extent, this required distinction between the
governing board of a public HSA and its separate governing body for health planning reflected Congress' view of
local elected officials as only one of many interest
groups that must be represented on an HSA's governing
body; to some extent, this requirement was a recognition
by Congress that the health system remained a predominantly
private operation;[18] and, to some extent, the governing
board/governing body distinction was a reaction to state
and local governmental lobbying.

Traditional participants in health policymaking resented
the involvement of state and local elected officials in
the development of the new planning law. Their past neglect of health planning efforts led congressional, HEW,
and health planning interests to consider their lobbying
with respect to health planning structure as a threat to
substantive health planning goals. Although these state
and local interests professed to support the goals of
health planning and to disagree only with its proposed
structure, supporters of a strengthened program tended
to see the two dimensions inextricably intertwined, each
dependent upon the other. Although elected officials
were able to secure in the new planning law a provision
allowing local governments and regional planning bodies
to be designated as HSAs, health planning advocates were
able to limit the number of such designations and to
curtail governmental control over planning agency operations where public HSAs were designated.

Governmental interest groups viewed the governing
board/governing body distinction as undermining the victory
they had won on the House floor when Congressman Moss succeeded in amending the House bill to permit public agency
designation as HSAs. The House health subcommittee had
been particularly unreceptive to the points raised by
these groups,[19] and the Moss amendment in the House over-
shadowed the fact that the Senate version of the planning
bill required public HSAs to establish a separate governing
body with exclusive authority to perform the functions of
a health planning agency. The House/Senate conference
committee accepted the Senate provision in this area, and
local governmental interests attempted to remedy the situation by arranging for colloquies to take place on the
House and Senate floors before a final vote on the planning
bill.

Dialogues took place between Senators Javits and Kennedy
on December 19, 1974, and between Congressmen Matsunaga
and Rogers on December 20, 1974. (Kennedy and Rogers
chaired the Senate and House health subcommittees that had
drafted the planning bill, and they were its chief supporters.) The dialogues were intended to soften the
language of the new planning bill and the conference
committee report that accompanied it by creating a public
record that the principal advocates of health planning
in the Congress agreed that the new bill gave the public
governing board of an HSA certain responsibilities over
the private governing body for health planning. In
response to questioning, Senator Kennedy and Congressman
Rogers agreed: that the private governing body for health
planning would be appointed and subject to removal by the
HSA's public governing board; that the private governing
body would be subject to the laws and regulations of the
public governing board; that, in carrying out its statutory
responsibilities, the private governing body would be subject to the rules and rulings of the public board; and
that the plans developed by the private governing body
would be submitted to the public parent agency for approval.
In each of these areas, the statements of Kennedy and Rogers
misrepresented the planning bill as drafted.

State and local governmental interest groups, especially
the National Association of Counties (NACo), approached
the HEW regulations-development process confidently. As
HEW began the considerable task of implementing the
planning law in early 1975, these groups had two key weapons
in their arsenal: (1) the language of the House and
Senate colloquies; and (2) the influence of Congressman
Moss, who threatened to focus the attention of his oversight subcommittee on health planning. NACo, whose members
stood to profit most from increased discretion for HSA
governing boards, directed the governmental lobby's efforts
to transfer the language of the House and Senate colloquies
into the HSA regulations that HEW was preparing. Congressman
Moss, for his part, made it perfectly clear that oversight
hearings would commence if the HSA regulations did not
properly reflect the colloquies.

Prompt implementation of the planning law was the chief
concern of Gene Rubel, whose Bureau of Health Planning and
Resources Development was charged with developing the regulations and providing the national direction for the new
planning system. He understood that lobbying and congressional oversight hearings regarding the new health

planning structure would only slow that process. Rubel
was familiar with the positions taken by the state and
local governmental lobby, but he shared the preference of
most congressional health subcommittee members and
staff for structuring a health planning system at the local
level that would not be dominated by any interest or
faction, including local elected officials. Rubel saw
merit in the intergovernmental and public/private checks
and balances set forth in Public Law 93-641, and he was
outspoken in his views. However, Rubel felt that designating and funding new state and local health planning
agencies should not be delayed due to the governing board/
governing body issue, and, after a great deal of contact
with and pressure from NACo representatives, he came to
favor including the meaning of the House and Senate colloquies in the HSA regulations.

Rubel estimated that the number of public agencies
that were willing and able to surmount the statutory and
procedural impediments to HSA designation would not be
large,[20] and he was persuaded that these agencies, having
proven their interest in health planning by surmounting
the impediments, should be afforded the degree of control
over the private governing body for health planning that
they sought.[21] Rubel became convinced that state and
local government groups, especially NACo, would not drop
the issue[22] and that Congressman Moss would, in fact, conduct oversight hearings on the planning law if the HSA
regulations were not written to his satisfaction.[23]
Finally, Rubel and others within HEW were impressed that,
from the beginning, NACo had directed the governmental
interest group efforts in this area in a pragmatic way.
They felt that NACo had resisted what must have been a
strong impulse to press simply for repeal of the national
health planning law. Instead, NACo had pressed for a
specific remedy to a situation about which it had strong
opinions. By adopting this strategy (targeting its opposition to the new law and demonstrating its understanding
of health policymaking by exploiting the support of Congressman Moss and by pressing for concrete regulatory
language), NACo gained entry to the regulations-development
process and the backing of HEW program officials.[24]

Opposition within HEW to Rubel and the NACo position
on the governing board/governing body relationship was
intense. The Office of the Assistant Secretary for Planning and Evaluation and the Office of the General Counsel
opposed writing HSA regulations following the course of

the House and Senate colloquies.[25] Nevertheless, the HSA
regulations, which were published in proposed form in the
Federal Register on October 17, 1975, granted public HSA
governing boards virtually total control over the governing bodies for health planning. As Rubel explained in an
interview, "We are bending over backwards in our regulations to accommodate them [state and local interest groups]
within the framework of the law."[26] The proposed rules
accommodated NACo's suggestions to the extent that HEW
found them to be legally supportable; however, to the
extent that the proposed rules did accommodate NACo, they
provoked countervailing pressure from congressional
health subcommittee sponsors of the health planning legislation and from the hospital industry.[27]

Congressmen Rogers and Hastings, in a letter to HEW
dated November 14, 1975, argued that the proposed rules
"are in conflict with the requirements of the law and
the legislative intent" regarding the relative powers of
the HSA governing board and governing body. The Rogers/
Hastings letter focused on the HSA's budget and emphasized
that the planning law and its legislative history "contain
no authority for giving the regular governing body [i.e.,
the public governing board] control over the HSA's budget."
The letter concluded that: "this provision . . . should
be deleted and complete control of the budget left with
the governing body for health planning."[28] The American
Hospital Association went even further, opposing governing
board involvement in framing the governing body's personnel policies, in setting the agency's operating procedures,
and in reviewing proposed actions of the governing body,
in addition to its role in setting the HSA's budget. The
AHA said that governing board performance of these functions, "if taken advantage of by the governmental parent
body, would seriously undermine the capacity of the HSA
governing body to conduct an effective areawide health
planning program and to develop as a strong local force."[29]

HEW officials found themselves in a most difficult position with respect to the governing board/governing body
issue in the final HSA regulations. In the House of Representatives, the chairman and the ranking minority member
of the health subcommittee were displeased that the proposed rules did not follow that they considered to be congressional intent, and, concurrently, the chairman of the
health oversight subcommittee was preparing to hold hearings
to demand that the public governing board be assigned power
over the private governing body for health planning greater

than even the proposed regulations permitted. Further,
medical and governmental interest groups were severely
opposed to one another on the issue,[30] and the arguments
for and against public control of the local planning
process were increasingly polarizing local planners,
governmental officials and community leaders, and medical
interests at the state and local levels.[31]

Public control over governing body activities in the
area of HSA budgets was eventually cut back somewhat in
the final HSA regulations that were published on March
26, 1976, due, in large part, to an opinion from HEW's
Office of the General Counsel.[32] Though HEW Secretary
Mathews accepted his department's legal advice on the
governing board/governing body issue, he took a public
position personally against the content of the final
regulations promulgated in his name. He remarked in
the preamble to the regulations that they "will engender
disabling conflict." Stating that the language of the
planning statute prevented him from resolving the issue
completely to governmental interest group satisfaction,
Mathews expressed his hope that the planning statute
would be rewritten on this point.[33] HEW supported NACo's
position in the final HSA regulations to the extent it
legally could, and it put a halt to lobbying on the
matter by the position it took in the preamble to those
regulations. HEW parted with the bulk of health planning
supporters in the Congress, in medical interest groups,
and among planners at the local level by agreeing to support the local governmental lobby's position when amendments to the planning law were considered. However,
a readjustment of HEW's position in the final HSA regulations concerning the governing board's control over the
governing body's budget demonstrated a certain responsiveness to the concerns of Congressmen Rogers and Hastings.
Mathews' decision to call for a legislative change to the
statute ended the administrative policymaking process with
respect to the public accountability of HSAs and effectively
shifted the issue back to the Congress and the courts for
further resolution.

Administrative Flexibility

State and local interest group arguments in support of
increased state flexibility in establishing and operating
State Health Planning and Development Agencies (SHPDAs)
and in administering certificate-of-need programs were

not as successful as those put forward in behalf of
increased public accountability at the substate regional
level. Although both congressional sponsors of health
planning and HEW officials were more inclined to respond
to gubernatorial concerns than to those raised by local
governmental officials, they were surprised by the gener-
ality of the arguments put forward by the governors'
Washington representatives.[34] National Governors' Conference objections to the new planning program since 1974
had been for the most part a general condemnation of
the shift in the planning law away from the new federalism,
and they had neglected specific commentary on (or commitment toward) the substantive goals of health planning.
During the legislative process, when the state governmental
lobby had objected to specific provisions in the planning
bills, there had been change. For example, state health
planning efforts were required to be conducted by an agency selected by the governor, not by an independent commission as had been originally proposed. Further, in response
to state lobbying, certain states were excepted from the
statute's requirement to establish substate health planning districts and to launch new local health planning
agencies. Nevertheless, it became clear to state governmental groups, especially the National Governors' Conference, that most local planning agencies would be private
nonprofit in sponsorship and that HSAs would compete with
state government for public acceptance on matters of state
health policy. Governmental interest group lobbyists and
certain governors called first for repeal and later for
amendment of the new law as they became aware that it
contained detailed requirements for SHPDAs and, perhaps
worst of all, that the new law afforded the HEW secretary
almost limitless discretion with respect to these state
agencies.

State governments, the level of government traditionally
responsible for the delivery and the regulation of health
care, were required by Public Law 93-641 to meet national
standards in health planning and regulation. This shift
in power fostered among states an increased mistrust
and resentment of the federal government, a belief that
the national government's new federalism relationship with
the states had been betrayed, and a determination to secure
from HEW the preferential treatment and deference that
had been denied them by Congress in the national health
planning law. Most state and local elected officials
tended to conclude that, by enacting the national health

planning law, "Congress has chosen to exclude elected
state and local government from health planning and
policy making," and they feared that the new health planning structure shifted "much of the responsibility for
health policy from government to cartel-like health systems agencies."[35] States retained the power to make
final decisions under the regulatory and other review
programs mandated by the new law, but most congressional
sponsors and HEW officials felt that the real keystone
to the health planning effort would be the health systems
agency.[36] State governmental lobbyists objected most to
what they termed "the OEO [Office of Economic Opportunity]
model applied to health" (i.e., the nongovernmental and
unaccountable private nonprofit character of local planning).[37] In addition, they protested the absence of
federal financial incentives (as well as the prominent
inclusion of severe financial penalties) in the health
planning law, the increased power of the HEW secretary
(and of the director of HEW's health planning bureau who
would act for the secretary) in relationship to state
officials, the intergovernmental conflict and competition
that would result from the HEW/SHPDA/HSA planning structure, and the general treatment in Public Law 93-641
of states as "poor, illiterate stepchildren, when in
fact several states have done far more to regulate health
costs on a long term basis than the federal government."[38]
The complaints were philosophical and diffused, and they
were provoked more by the provisions of the planning law
than specific HEW action.

Washington-based groups representing state and local
elected officials tended to support one another during
the process of implementing Public Law 93-641, but, as
NACo had taken the lead in lobbying for concessions in
the HSA regulations, the National Governors' Conference
(NGC) served as the chief advocate of a strengthened state
role in the new health planning/regulation system. NGC
did not approach HEW with a detailed understanding of the
new law or with specific language that it sought to include
in administrative regulations. Rather, on February 19,
1975, NGC's Committee on Human Resources took a public
position on the new law, finding it "completely unacceptable
in its lack of clear lines of public accountability," and
urging that state governors (instead of the HEW secretary)
be given complete control over state and local health
planning. The Committee on Human Resources did not distinguish between HEW and the Congress in making these demands,

and this action only served to weaken the argument for an increased state role in health planning. Although NGC professed to disagree only with the administrative structure (and not the regulatory goals) of the new planning law, its failure to demonstrate a substantive understanding of health planning and a working knowledge of the new law reinforced HEW's suspicion that state politicians might undermine the planning process. Indeed, much of the early NGC/HEW relationship was devoted to clarifying for governors and their representatives the requirements of the law. Much of this task fell to Gene Rubel, who directed HEW's health planning effort. To the extent that Rubel's own support of the planning law was apparent (he did not try in the least to mask it), gubernatorial opposition to the planning law became directed toward him. Soon, NGC, led by Washington Governor Daniel J. Evans and Idaho Governor Cecil D. Andrus, had two goals with respect to the national health planning program: (1) prompt amendment of the planning law; and (2) removal of Rubel as the HEW official responsible for implementing the planning program.

NGC did not succeed in amending the planning law. Although Senator Magnuson introduced amendments prepared by Governor Evans on June 10, 1975, their reception by the Congress was markedly cool. Nevertheless, state officials called for hearings on the proposed amendments, which would give the HEW secretary the power to grant waivers to the provisions of Public Law 93-641 that the governmental lobby found objectionable. These waivers would undermine the planning structure that congressional sponsors felt was essential to the success of the new program. Health planning supporters in HEW and Congress understood that hearings would only delay the new planning law's implementation and would permit medical interest groups, especially the American Medical Association, the chance to cut back its regulatory provisions.[39] Therefore, Congressman Rogers and Senator Kennedy dismissed the governors' proposal for amendments in a letter written to each governor. The Rogers/Kennedy letter ended the NGC's hope for a change in the statutory ground rules for health planning in 1975, and it brought the NGC to realize the importance of the HEW regulations-development process.

The regulations governing state health planning agencies were developed by HEW program staff in an atmosphere that favored granting states as much flexibility as the planning statute permitted.[40] The new HEW secretary, David Mathews,

was interested in accommodating the NGC concerns to the
extent legally permissible, and the statute already contained much of the detail normally found in administrative
regulation. Beyond this, Rubel was not intimidated by
state governmental lobbying, and he saw the interest of
state governors as having substantial benefits for the
planning program. Rubel felt that the statute might be
sufficiently offensive to the governors that it would
provoke them to support state health planning as a
defense against possible HEW intrusion into state affairs
and HSA competition for public acceptance and legitimacy.
In this way, one of the chief reasons for the failure
of the comprehensive health planning program would be overcome.[41] Thus, Rubel was committed toward the intergovernmental rivalries and conflicts generated by the new
health planning structure. The state government lobby
preferred instead an ordered HEW/SHPDA/HSA relationship
with a controlling role for the state. To a large extent,
Rubel's commitment toward intergovernmental conflict under-
lay NGC pressure for Rubel's removal as HEW's health
planning director. On August 29, 1975, Governor Andrus,
chairman of NGC's Human Resources Committee, asked
Rubel's direct superior, Dr. Kenneth Endicott, for new
leadership of the planning program. In March 1976, after
regulations governing state health planning had been published in the *Federal Register* in proposed form, Rubel
was pressured into resigning as acting director of the
health planning program.

While there was a great deal of mistrust and antagonism
between NGC and HEW in the months following enactment of
the national health planning law, both tried to develop
working relationships with one another. In late May 1975,
the NGC developed a proposal to form a consortium of
states to address the problems associated with establishing and operating new state health planning agencies.[42]
The proposal was funded by HEW, and while there was some
ambiguity regarding the real task of the consortium (NGC
felt that the consortium should provide advice to HEW
with respect to the planning law's implementation, and
HEW expected the consortium to provide advice to the
states concerning ways to meet the specifications of
Public Law 93-641), both NGC and HEW were convinced of
its merit. For state governors and their representatives,
the consortium served two functions: (1) it provided a
vehicle for state officials to gain the background regarding health planning and Public Law 93-641 necessary
to develop and press for reasonable concessions in HEW

regulations; and (2) it provided through the meetings of
the consortium a good deal of HEW program staff exposure
to state officials and the problems associated with administering health planning at the state level. Over
time, state officials and HEW program staff grew to
understand and to sympathize with one another's legal
and organizational constraints, and they began to
anticipate each other's needs.

NGC's Health Planning Consortium was continued and expanded in size in February 1976, under a new contract with
HEW's Health Planning Bureau, and it continued to challenge
the assumption NGC saw underlying Public Law 93-641, "that
there is one 'best' planning structure and methodology."[43]
State understanding of health planning increased during
the course of this contract, and, as NGC recommendations
became more specific and its familiarity with the substantive goals of Public Law 93-641 grew, gubernatorial
staff/HEW program staff relationships became quite
cordial. Although NGC's final report for this contract
reiterated its position advocating HEW/SHPDA/HSA cooperation (instead of conflict) and a strong coordinating role
for the states, the report evidenced a significant advance in understanding HEW's predicament in administering
a highly specific statute under close congressional scrutiny,
and it moderated its criticism of HEW by recognizing where
distinct amendments to Public Law 93-641 would permit HEW
the discretion to grant states the administrative flexibility with respect to planning structure that they desired. Further, the consortium report indicated a growing
interest in and grasp of the regulatory purpose of the
health planning law. This development, more than any other,
drew support from HEW program staff for NGC suggestions.
Where it became clear that state officials were committed
to the substantive goals of health planning, HEW saw
justification for giving states the administrative flexibility they desired.

NGC attention was focused primarily on the organizational
requirements for state health planning agencies. HEW
responsiveness in this area was not particularly difficult,
since the statute was already quite detailed and since
there was little prospect of statutory change in the near
future. With respect to the federal standards for state
certificate-of-need programs, however, NGC interest in
the procedural (as opposed to the substantive) elements
of state regulatory programs permitted federal program
staff wide latitude in the regulations-development process.

Although the national health planning law was fairly
specific on the procedures that SHPDAs must follow in
administering regulatory and other review programs,
the statute did grant the HEW secretary the power to
permit exceptions (or waivers) to them.[44] Thus, state
officials could press HEW for individual treatment and
sensitivity to unique state conditions in this area.
The planning law allowed in this area what NGC had sought
in other areas from Congress in 1975 without success. NGC
and gubernatorial representatives, however, remained preoccupied by the procedural standards for state certificate-
of-need programs. To HEW officials, procedural noncompliance by a state with the federal certificate-of-need
standards would not result in the withholding of funds
that was called for in the planning law--the HEW secretary
could grant a procedural exception to prevent the situation
from arising. Rather, the key issues before HEW program
staff concerned the extent of state regulation (i.e., the
range of facilities subject to review) and the stringency
of state regulation (i.e., the precise activities or
thresholds that would initiate the review process). The
planning law gave only broad direction in the matter, and
the absence of a state governmental position on this
issue conditioned officials throughout HEW to expect
prompt state implementation of whatever federal regulatory
standards were developed.[45]

NGC views were conspicuously absent from internal
HEW discussions on the scope of coverage that would be
required in federal regulations governing state certificate-
of-need programs. Even though the points of program coverage for state certificate-of-need programs being developed
by HEW program staff would eventually need to be included
in state statutes and regulations, and even though federal
standards could be changed (and even expanded) in the
future, NGC and state governors did not actively lobby
with respect to them. In the late 1970s, when Public Law
93-641 required the imposition of financial penalties upon
states out of compliance with federal health planning requirements, the major reasons for state noncompliance were
the substantive (not the procedural) provisions of the
federal certificate-of-need regulations. As each state
grappled with the cumbersome process of securing authoriza-
tions from state legislatures and drafting state implementing
regulations, it generally did so alone, with little advice
or support from NGC, the Health Planning Consortium, or
other states.

As HEW officials attempted to set in place the structural requirements for the new health planning system, and as they attempted to manage the issues raised by state and local elected officials, they were simultaneously dealing with the claims raised by medical interest groups. Medical group reactions to the planning law were far from uniform, ranging from general acceptance to outright hostility. Their participation in the administrative policymaking process was stimulated by the regulatory potential of the new law, and the vague wording of the substantive (or regulatory) portions of the planning statute underscored the importance of the federal regulations that were being developed. With the exception of the posture assumed by the American Medical Association, which sought to block implementation of the planning law through court action, medical interest group lobbying was continuous and intense. HEW officials had anticipated this action, and the administrative policymaking process was distinguished more by the number of top HEW officials participating in it than by the way in which issues were resolved. However, while state and local governmental interest groups limited their involvement in the HEW regulations-development process to organizational and procedural matters, medical interest groups did not confine their attention to any one aspect of the planning law.

Like congressional supporters of health planning and HEW officials, representatives of medical groups considered the structural provisions of the health planning law to be of equal importance to its substantive provisions, and they tended to oppose arguments advanced by the governmental lobby in support of a controlling role for elected officials The representation requirements for HSA governing boards, the mandated relationships between HSAs and SHPDAs, and the amount of HEW involvement in state and local planning activities were issues that would have a strong impact on the regulatory activities of planning agencies. Medical interest group support of HEW's position on the structure of state and local health planning also aided them in their lobbying with respect to issues of program substance. Similarly, state and local governmental neglect of substantive issues hindered their attempts to shape the new planning structure.

In many respects, NGC and state governmental interests seemed to focus on planning procedure at the expense of regulatory substance, HEW leadership style at the expense of program content. State governmental interest in health

planning seemed to wane after the resignation of Gene
Rubel and to have reached a low point as individual states
faced their own deadlines for compliance with the planning
law's requirements. Indeed, by the time the Carter administration began drafting programs designed to expand
health regulation and build on state certificate-of-need
programs in preparation for a national health insurance
proposal, HEW's funding for the consortium had ended,
and NGC resources devoted to health issues had been cut
back to the level they had been (one staff person for
the entire human resources field) in the early 1970s.

CONCLUDING REMARKS

The years that followed the legislative enactment and
the development of the key regulations implementing Public
Law 93-641 did not produce the degree of intergovernmental
conflict that was anticipated by state and local governmental lobbyists (or intended by health planning supporters) in the mid-1970s. The congressional sponsors
of the new health planning law had hoped to establish
a system of checks and balances among the various levels
of government, as well as among the consumers, providers,
and local elected officials represented on HSA governing
boards. Instead, the state and local health planning
activities supported by Public Law 93-641 have been characterized by their diversity, their reflection of individual HSA/state agency relationships, and the lack of
federal policy direction. Federal administrators
of the health planning law have tended, for the most part,
to play a nondirective role toward state and local health
planning efforts, and the intergovernmental conflict and
cooperation that has occurred in health planning has been
less the result of provisions in federal statute and regulation than the result of unique local situations. Health
planning and regulation, once resisted by most medical and
governmental lobby groups as an intrusion into local affairs, has become an acceptable feature on the intergovernmental landscape. It is ironic that, as national
policymakers have searched for the means to extend the
amount of federal control over private health activities
in order to contain health costs, the structure of health
planning has come to represent the countervailing public
values of decentralization and deference to subnational
power centers (both public and private). This lack of

control over the day-to-day operations of health planning
had led top federal policymakers to discount the role of
health planning in contributing to their substantive (i.e.,
regulatory) goals for the health system.

NOTES

1. Quoted in John K. Iglehart, "Health Report/Stiff
Industry Regulations Likely; Congress, HEW Near Agreement,"
National Journal Reports VI(February 2, 1974), p. 164.
Congressman Roy became convinced of the need for expanded
health planning agency powers when he served on the board
of a comprehensive health planning agency in Topeka, Kansas.
Regarding this experience, Roy observed that: "While we
sat and talked about health planning one new hospital
was built and another expanded 40 percent in Topeka
and they were 400 yards apart." Quoted in John K. Iglehart, "Health Report/Executive-Congressional Coalition
Seeks Tighter Regulation for Medical-Services Industry,"
National Journal Reports V(November 10, 1973), p. 1692.
2. Congressman James F. Hastings related health planning decisions to the development of a national health insurance program when he stated during a hearing on the
various health planning proposals:

The various proposals before us took over a year
to develop, and the issues are many and complex.
The decisions we make during the next few weeks
on the questions of medical care resource planning,
development, and allocation will be central to any
program of national health insurance.

See U.S. Congress, House Committee on Interstate and
Foreign Commerce, Subcommittee on Public Health and Environment, *National Health Policy and Health Resources
Development,* Hearings on H.R. 12052, H.R. 12053, H.R.
13472, H.R. 13995, H.R. 14164, H.R. 14191, H.R. 14409,
and H.R. 14698, 93rd Congress, 2nd Session (Washington:
U.S. Government Printing Office, 1974), p. 391 (hereafter cited as House Subcommittee Hearings). See also
the Senate debate on the conference committee report on
S. 2994, the Senate version of the national health planning
law, in the December 19, 1974, *Congressional Record,*
p. S22258.

3. The proscription in the comprehensive health planning law against interference by the national government with the private practice of medicine was an extension of a congressional policy articulated in the Medicare statute (see the Social Security Act at section 1801). Section 1801 states that the federal government shall do nothing "to exercise control over the practice of medicine or the manner in which medical services are provided. . . ."

4. Certain of these factors are recognized by Drew Altman in his article, "The Politics of Health Care Regulation: The Case of the National Health Planning and Resources Development Act," *Journal of Health Politics, Policy and Law* II(Winter, 1978), pp. 560-580; see in particular p. 565.

5. The congressional health subcommittees may have had other reasons for drafting a very detailed bill. In other health program areas, the Nixon administration had cut back HEW's approach to categorical grants under the rubric of the new federalism, it had redirected some health programs toward administration-set goals which were contrary to congressional preferences, and it had even impounded congressional appropriations for purposes it considered to be inappropriate.

6. Interview, Eugene J. Rubel, former acting director, Bureau of Health Planning and Resources Development, U.S. Department of Health, Education, and Welfare, Washington, D.C., March 1 and 30, 1979. The congressional focus on administrative implementation is particularly evident in the conference report accompanying the compromise House/Senate health planning bill. The report described the bill's guidelines for designating new substate planning boundaries as "self executing." See U.S. Congress, House of Representatives, *National Health Planning and Resources Development Act of 1974,* Conference Report to accompany S. 2994, Report No. 93-1640, 93rd Congress, 2nd Session (Washington: U.S. Government Printing Office, December 19, 1974), p. 65.

7. William J. Curran, "Present at the Creation: Health Planning and the Inevitable Reorganization," *Health Care Management Review* I(Winter, 1976), p. 38.

8. The most vocal governmental interest groups included the National Governors' Conference (later renamed the National Governors' Association), the National Association of Counties, the National Association of Regional Councils, and the National League of Cities/United States Conference of Mayors.

9. "County Opinion: CHP," *County News*, National Association of Counties (September 9, 1974).
10. See U.S. Congress, House Committee on Interstate
and Foreign Commerce, *National Health Policy, Planning,
and Resources Development Act of 1974*, 93rd Congress, 2nd
Session (Washington: U.S. Government Printing Office,
1974), pp. 40-41.
11. Quoted in Iglehart, "Health Report/Stiff Industry
Regulations Likely . . .," p. 168.
12. Quoted in *Ibid.*, p. 166.
13. According to Dr. S. Philip Caper of Senator Edward
M. Kennedy's staff, disinclination to upgrade the state
role in health planning was the result of

. . . a general doubt of the ability of state
governments to deal in a complex area such as
this. They have administered the Medicaid program poorly, for example. Things that are complex
take a lot of administrative skill and talent and
states just have not shown that. [*Ibid.*, p. 167]

14. Interview, Rubel.
15. Steven Sieverts, *Health Planning Issues and Public
Law 93-641* (Chicago: American Hospital Association, 1977),
p. 12.
16. *Ibid.*, pp. 35-39.
17. Section 1512(b)(3)(A) of the Public Health Service
Act.
18. For example, in fiscal year 1975, the private sector generated 57.8 percent of the $118.5 billion in na-
tional health expenditures. See Iglehart, "HEW Takes
Final Step Down Road to Local Health Planning Network,"
National Journal VIII (April 3, 1976), p. 437.
19. Interview, Rubel.
20. Rubel estimated that approximately 20 percent of the
HSAs would be public agencies. Iglehart, "Health Report/
State, County Governments Win Key Roles in New Program,"
National Journal VII(November 8, 1975), p. 1534.
21. Interview, Rubel.
22. Rubel's attendance at NACo's annual convention on
June 22-25, 1975, marked a turning point in his approach
to the governing board/governing body issue. Iglehart,
"Health Report/State, County Governments Win Key Roles in
New Programs," p. 1536.
23. In an interview, Rubel stated that: "I concluded
that Moss was serious I agonized and finally said, 'okay,
let's see what we can work out'" with the county officials.
Ibid., p. 1537.

141

24. Interview, Rubel.
25. Iglehart, "Health Report/State, County Governments Win Key Roles in New Program," p. 1537.
26. Quoted in Iglehart, "Health Report/States, Cities Seek Role Over Regional Planning Bodies," *National Journal* VII(August 23, 1975), p. 1207.
27. John K. Iglehart, "Health Report/Key Legislators, Hospital Lobby Question Local Planning Role," *National Journal* VII(November 11, 1975), pp. 1641-1642.
28. Quoted in *Ibid.*, p. 1641.
29. Quoted in *Ibid.*, p. 1642. See also Steven Sieverts quoted in Iglehart, "Health Report/State, County Governments Win Key Roles in New Program," p. 1539.
30. See, for example, *Washington Report on Medicine and Health*, No. 1479 (November 3, 1975), p. 2.
31. See Anthony Robbins, "Who Should Make Public Policy for Health?" *American Journal of Public Health* LXVI (May, 1976), p. 431. See also the letters to the editor that this piece provoked in the *American Journal of Public Health* LXVI(October, 1976), pp. 1005-1007. For differing views on the role of the HSAs, see: Bruce C. Vladeck, "Interest-Group Representation and the HSAs: Health Planning and Political Theory," *American Journal of Public Health* LXVII(January, 1977), pp. 23-29; Steven Sieverts, "Issues in the Implementation of P.L. 93-641: The Preliminary Regulations and 'Public' Health Systems Agencies," paper presented at the Special Briefing Session on P.L. 93-641, sponsored by the U.S. Department of Health, Education, and Welfare and the National Health Council, Washington, D.C., October 28, 1975.
32. Iglehart, "HEW Takes Final Step Down Road to Local Health Planning Network," p. 437.
33. See the Preamble to the Final Rules governing "Health Systems Agencies," *Federal Register*, Vol. 41, No. 60 (March 26, 1976), p. 12812.
34. Interview, Rubel.
35. Robbins, p. 431.
36. See, for example, U.S. Congress, House Committee on Interstate and Foreign Commerce, *National Health Policy, Planning, and Resources Development Act of 1974*, 93rd Congress, 2nd Session (Washington: U.S. Government Printing Office, 1974), p. 52.
37. Kevin McKenna, Special Counsel to Governor Philip W. Noel of Rhode Island, quoted in House Subcommittee

Hearings, p. 588. In this same vein, Curran concluded that HSAs are "essentially Federal creatures, even though their primary activity is to be planning and development of local health services and facilities." See Curran, p. 40.

38. McKenna, quoted in House Subcommittee Hearings, p. 596.

39. Iglehart, "Health Report/States, Cities Seek Role Over Regional Planning Bodies," p. 1207.

40. Iglehart, "HEW Takes Final Step Down Road to Local Health Planning Network," p. 438.

41. Interview, Rubel.

42. See the Draft "Proposal for a Consortium of States to Develop Guidelines for the State Administrative Program," prepared by the National Governors' Conference, May 22, 1975.

43. Health Planning Consortium, National Governors' Conference, *Making the National Health Planning Law Work: The State Perspective* (Washington: Center for Policy Research and Analysis, National Governors' Conference, February, 1977), p. v.

44. Section 1532(a) of the Public Health Service Act.

45. Throughout the process of implementing Public Law 93-641, HEW officials consistently downplayed the problems that would arise in securing state compliance (through enactment of new state legislation, amendment of existing state legislation, and the development of administrative regulations) in order to meet federal standards.

BOTTOMS UP IS UPSIDE DOWN

Harvey M. Sapolsky

*Control of much of the health care industry's
capital expenditures rests, today, with the health
planning agencies. In this paper, Sapolsky points
out some of the problems and contradictions in the
current situation. Sapolsky proposes an alternative
system, with two key elements--first, a congres-
sionally determined capital expenditure limit, and
second, allocation of capital resting squarely in
the hands of payors and of consumers.*

The Founding Fathers believed in democracy. They created
a union of sovereign states to fight the tyranny of a
distant, royalist power. They sought to establish institutions responsive to the popular will. And they encouraged
individuals to participate in the governance of their own
society.

The Founding Fathers, however, also believed in effective government. When the Articles of Confederation, which
formed the union, were demonstrated to be unworkable, they
drafted the Constitution to preserve both individual
liberty and governmental authority. Liberty was protected
in the Bill of Rights, while the passion of majorities
was constrained through a division of powers among the
branches of government and between the states and the
national government. And, the Founding Fathers were wise
enough to design a flexible Constitution, one capable of
adjusting to changing conditions.

They, of course, were not blessed with total foresight.
They had no intimation of the wonders of modern medicine.
They did not contemplate the uses of a CT scanner, let

143

alone the design of a system to allocate them among the nation's hospitals. They were not familiar with terms such as lease back, contract management, batching, and maxicap. And, no one of them thought that the descendants of John Hancock would be selling health insurance.

It was our choice, not the Founding Fathers', as to how the health planning system should be organized. But like them, we ought to be willing to admit and correct the mistakes we have made in designing governmental arrangements. Perhaps we were diverted by the Watergate crisis or perhaps we were misled by well-organized lobbies when we chose the present for health planning in 1974.[1] Whatever the cause of our errors, it should be obvious to us that there is need now to redesign completely the health planning system.

REPRESENTATION WITHOUT TAXATION

When the good citizens of Boston assembled in Indian disguise to throw the crates of tea into the harbor, they were protesting an arbitrarily imposed tax. The British government had taxed tea without giving those who were to pay the tax an opportunity to participate in decisions determining the need for and the uses of the revenues expected. In organizing our current health planning system, we have committed a similar injustice, giving effective representation to all except those who pay the costs the system can impose. Providers and consumers of health care are adequately represented in the system, but not the premium and rate payors. The injustice is compounded by the insistence that the representation be locally based and largely nongovernmental. It is a formula for irresponsible behavior.

Health care costs are determined locally, but are paid for the most part in broader jurisdictions. Direct out-of-pocket payments by individuals account for only 30 percent of health care expenditures (and considerably less of hospital expenditures) with the remainder divided between government, both state and local, and insurance mechanisms. Federal payments are derived from Social Security and general taxes, rates that are obviously set nationally. The state contribution, primarily for Medicaid, is the result of taxes imposed statewide. Blue Cross/Blue Shield premium rates are determined either for geographic areas larger than individual communities or on the basis of group experience. Private insurance carrier premiums most often reflect companywide (state, regional, or national) experience for group purchases, not local costs.[2]

Health care costs, however, are the product of locally based resources and locally determined efficiencies. A community with high rates of medical service utilization, lots of hospital beds, many specialists, and a medical school or two will have higher health care costs than an equally populous community with fewer sophisticated facilities and personnel and lower utilization rates. Thus, while the costs for health services in Cleveland reflect the services available in Cleveland, the financing of these services is shared with the citizens of Toledo, Akron, Peoria, Salt Lake City, and everywhere else in the country, an arrangement surely not encouraging of local restraints.

No comfort can be found in the fact that some local planning councils have occasionally shown a willingness to limit the availability of local health services, especially if it involves the entry of new competition. The federal government has labored hard to convince local consumers, particularly those serving on planning councils, that the interests of consumers were other than those demanded by the logic of structure in which they function. Moreover, local health care providers often see benefit in opposing capital investments proposed by potential rivals.[3] But, in the end, laggard communities are certain to realize that the health care resources they acquire are largely paid for by others though these resources serve only themselves.

BEGGAR THY NEIGHBOR

The organizations representing health care payors are an incohesive lot. Numbering in the thousands, they show no inclination to cooperate. The private insurers among them compete for the same clients and differ considerably in size and organizational structure with some being profit makers, while others are not for profit. The public agencies financing health care services mistrust each other and the private health insurers. Most of them stand as potential claimants for a dominant role in the administration of national health insurance if such a program were to be adopted. Although all are victims of the localism besetting health care services in the United

States, they have not formed a common front to gain control of the planning system. Instead, they seek advantage over one another in the financing of health services. And, in the process, dissipate their inherent collective strength.[4]

The federal government finds comfort in the multitude of accounting and payment regulations it issues. It avoids, for example, paying a full share of hospital malpractice and bad debt claims. It also reduces its obligations by limiting the charges hospitals are permitted for routine services to federal beneficiaries. All of which adds to the cost of other health care payors.

State governments are even more notorious for their attempts to pass on the costs to others. Altering the standards for Medicaid eligibility has been one of their favorite devices. Another has been to pay vendors late, sometimes years late, in the hope that the vendors will accept less than full payment or not press claims. Such practices antagonize providers, but the fewer providers willing to accept state paid patients, the lower the cost of health services are likely to be to the states.[5]

Blue Cross and Blue Shield, because of the historic ties to health care providers, often obtain significant discounts in service charges. Private insurers have countered this technique by offering group clients premiums based on their individual experience--a practice now adopted by Blue Cross and Blue Shield plans as well. Health Maintenance Organizations reduce their risks by searching out client populations that are young, healthy, and mobile and thus that are likely to have low utilization of services.[6]

Each organization seeks self-protection, but at the expense of the others. Without cooperation among the payors, however, their efforts are largely in vain. Costs are passed among the payors of health services in a cycle of adjustment-counter adjustment that prevents an achievement of permanent advantage on the part of any one of them or the exercise of effective countervailing power against the providers of health care services.

CHAINS OF CIRCUMSTANCE

The localism of the planning system and the disunity of the payors give strength to the providers of health services. The fastest growing phenomenon within the

health sector is the growth of hospital chains. In recent
years, hundreds of hospitals have become participants
in chains through management contracts, acquisitions, or
direct memberships. There are for-profit chains, nonprofit
chains, Protestant chains, and Catholic chains. Investor-
owned chains alone account for 10 percent of the nation's
supply of hospital beds. No better buy exists on the stock
exchange than the listed firms. And, as the purchasers of
this stock know, their attraction lies largely in their
ability to foil the regulators.[7]

To be sure, other arguments are advanced for the growth
of chains. Economies can be achieved in the group purchase of supplies. Manufacturers willingly compete for
the business of chains by offering volume discounts.
Centralized inventories can be maintained to bolster
purchase orders. There also may be internal economies to
be gained. Chains are likely to be more able to hire and
train skilled administrators than are individual hospitals,
as they offer better career advancement opportunities.
They can compare performance across hospitals and dis-
seminate quickly improved methods among affiliates. Hospitals need no longer be dependent upon the managerial
abilities of local trustees, employees, and physicians.

But the chains offer a more important advantage: centralized management can easily play one set of regulators
against another. Built largely from preexisting hospitals,
the chains know that the planning system protects established providers best. Any new investments desired can
be placed in the most favorable jurisdictions. Prices
and services can be structured to exploit differences in
policies among reimbursement agencies and insurers.
Proposals for expansion can be prepared and defended by
experienced specialists serving the entire chain. There
are also profits to be made in real estate transactions
timed to take advantage of loopholes in regulations.

As the chains grow, so will their political influence.
Already, the association of proprietary hospitals, the
Federation of American Hospitals, holds equal standing
with the American Hospital Association in the formulation of congressional legislation.[8] Although they are
regional and national in scope, the chains are champions
of local initiatives in health care planning, the so-called
bottoms up approach to planning. It could not be otherwise, however, as the chains draw sustenance from the fact
that they need now only cope with a highly fragmented
system of regulation.

BEGGAR THY NATION

Decisions to invest in health care capital, the prime focus
of the planning system, are but the final steps in a
series of decisions that determine future health care
expenditures. Health care capital embodies new technologies and requires specialized manpower for its utilization. The availability of new techniques and trained
personnel produces enormous pressure to invest in facilities and equipment and yet, decisions affecting the development of medical technologies and the training of
medical specialists are made independently of the planning
system and with little concern as to their effect on the
costs of health services.

Although the federal government heavily subsidizes
**both medical research and the training of medical special-
ists, it provides but the mildest directional guidance**
to either enterprise. The medical research community
largely governs itself, receiving its allocations by
disease categories and then converting them to fit the
preference of its constituent disciplines. The specific
topics to be pursued are the choice of individual investi-
gators subject to peer pressure and review. Entrepreneur-
ial initiative, aided by venture capital and federal contracts, brings the results of research to an eager and
rich market. Medical educators seemingly are more tightly
bound as they are dependent upon less widely available
training grants. Skillful tapping of the various medical
service reimbursement systems, however, can usually provide them with the desired degree of financial independence. The types of training programs actually mounted
then depend upon the ambition of individual educators and
the institutions to which they are affiliated. To the
extent it does exist in the United States, planning for
research and training is thus only a minor variant of the
decentralized decision-making arrangements prevalent in
the facility planning system, the revered bottoms up
variety of planning.[9]

The health system consequences of decisions produced
by such arrangements, however, are enormous. Consider
the case of the totally implantable artificial heart program. A gleam in the eyes of a handful of researchers two
decades ago, it now stands at the threshold of completion.
To date, less than $200 million have been expended with
annual increments rarely exceeding $10 million. But
once the device has been perfected, as surely it will,

the cost of providing them for even a modest patient
population will involve the expenditure of billions upon
billions of dollars and demand the attention of hundreds
of surgical teams and thousands of specialized personnel.
At no time in the history of the program, however, have
the benefits of alternative uses of similar-sized resource
commitments been compared to those of the artificial
heart. Instead, the program was judged on the basis of
its research promise and its impact on the budgets of the
granting agencies.[10]

To expect serious evaluations of system implications
will occur when the heart is perfected is to expect too
much from any assembly of decision-makers. At that time
the decisions will be affecting what Thomas Shelling has
called individual lives as opposed to statistical lives.
A heart in the hand will always be implanted; rationing
caused by shortages will not be tolerated. The opportunity to consider alternatives comes only at the initial
stages of investigation.

With the government absorbing an ever increasing share
of health care expenditures, and with these expenditures
increasing rapidly, government cannot responsibly continue
to permit scientists and educators to determine the scale
and content of health care services. Attempts to confine
governmental controls to the construction and renewal of
facilities are inevitably frustrated by citizen demands
to have convenient access to the best-available care.
It is inevitable that government will seek to define
what services are to be available through controls imposed upon medical research and training.[11] For it to
do otherwise would be to delegate permanent control of
a significant portion of public expenditures to self-
governing professions.

THE DOLLAR VOTE

Of course, if individuals were to pay directly a significant share of their own health care costs, there would
be little need for government to be concerned about what
therapies doctors utilized or how many beds a particular
hospital had. The truly enfranchised consumer, one made
financially responsible for his or her choices, would
add the missing element of self-restraint to the utilization of health services. A variety of proposals have

been advanced recently to achieve this apparently happy
state of a disciplined democracy in health care.

The fatal flaw in these proposals, however, is their
failure to appreciate the extent to which subsidies inter-
lace the market for health care services. Not only are
the poor and the elderly subsidized, but so too are parents, urban dwellers, Easterners, Indians, veterans, employees of most large firms, and the unscrupulous. The
subsidized cannot be expected to surrender gracefully
their privileges. The subsidizers lack the will to force
the issue. In fact, the subsidies are so prevalent in
the society that few should want to risk their full reve-
lation lest an unknown but real benefit be jeopardized.

No one should forget the origins of these subsidies.
The fears that illness, disease, and injury evoke make us
wish to have always adequate resources at hand for our
own care. Equity considerations drive us to be concerned
about those financially less fortunate than ourselves.
Theoretical doctrines about the virtues of freely functioning markets cannot eliminate these fears and values.

Given that the implementation of promarket proposals
would subject the provision of health services to the rig-
ors of competition, one might suspect that health care
providers would be their strongest opponents. But such
is not the case. Instead, there are ringing endorsements
from provider associations, adding political credence to
the proposals' substantial intellectual appeal. Cynics,
however, may wonder about the sincerity of the endorsements for the longer market type solutions hold the stage,
the longer is delayed the adoption of reforms that involve
the imposition of greater governmental controls.

THINKING ABOUT THE UNTHINKABLE

Strangely missing from consideration are specifications
as to how effective controls might be structured. Perhaps some think that there is no such thing as effective
controls and thus see no purpose in making the effort.
Or perhaps some think that provider opposition to controls
is so great that their adoption is highly unlikely and
thus that any effort at specification is wasteful. But
unless there is a set of controls to examine, there can
be no debate on the merits or the political acceptability
of controls. Let me be the boldest (or the most fool-
hardy) and offer a proposal.

Investments in health care facilities and technologies
are not in themselves socially undesirable. The health
care sector, like any other, needs to replace its worn-
out, obsolete, and mislocated plant and equipment. There
are even arguments to be made on the necessity of adding
to the capital stock. Worthwhile innovations do occur.
Rather, the problem lies in the divergence that might
develop between interests of providers and consumers, on
one hand, and the interests of society, on the other, in
the allocation of capital within the sector.

The interests of providers are apparently well served
by the current pattern of health care investments. Whether
generated by profit, prestige, or the perversities of the
reimbursement systems, these investments emphasize acute
care and sophisticated technologies while neglecting ambulatory care, preventive medicine, and long-term care.
The only complaints heard from providers are those voiced
when a certificate-of-need agency denies their investment
application or endorses that of a rival. Consumers, with
rare exceptions, remain content in a web of subsidies,
unconcerned or uninformed about opportunities foregone.

Less clear is how well the current pattern of investment serves society's interests. There is neither a single forum where these interests are articulated nor any
attempt to reconcile them when they are expressed. Local
agencies review proposals for health care projects, but
are divorced from the responsibilities of paying for the
health services that approved projects generate. National agencies provide grants and other forms of assistance
for the provision of certain types of services, but have
little influence over their location and essentially none
over their quality. Decisions affecting the federal
government's substantial investments in health care research are made independently of their likely future impact on the health care delivery system. No one, except
perhaps the providers, seems to know or care much about
the long-term implications of any particular investment
that expands or renews existing service capacity.

Societal interests can, of course, be in conflict.
Such would seem to be the case with regard to public
attitudes toward the performance of the health care sector. There is concern about the rising cost of health
care services, but also concern about the quality and
accessibility of these services. Given the absence of
effective market forces, what is needed are arrangements
to ensure that these interests are fully expressed and
balanced against one another.

Congress, as the political system's most representative
and responsive body, should hold responsibility for deciding the levels of investment to be permitted each year
in major categories of health care capital, e.g., acute
care, nursing homes, ambulatory care, and thus the total
to be invested annually in the health care sector. The
administration would advise the Congress on the desira-
bility of alternative levels of investments in each category of capital. It would also prepare and defend proposals for the location of licensing authority by each category. Presumably some categories would be reserved for
central licensing, perhaps new hospital beds and the most
major acute care equipment, while others might be delegated to regional or state levels such as nursing home
beds and hospital renovation. The Congress would modify
and approve these proposals.

For each category, a board would be established at the
designated level. The boards would be composed of representatives of health care payors and consumers, but not
providers. The payors would hold a majority and their
seats would be allocated according to the percentages of
services for which they provided reimbursement in the
appropriate category. In most instances, governments,
both federal and state, would hold dominant influence as
they are the dominant payors, but other payors representing
the group and individual purchasers of health care services would also be present to express their interests.
The consumers could be appointed by the Congress on nomina-
tion by the President according to party label, as are
the members of other regulatory agencies. This would
ensure responsible and responsive representation of consumer interests.

The boards would prepare criteria for the award of
construction or equipment purchase licenses, which they
would then award up to the limit approved by Congress on
application by current or potential providers. Federal,
state, and local government providers would also have to
compete for the available licenses in each category of
investment. The Congress could review and alter the criteria the boards prepare. Executive agencies and the
public would have the opportunity in open hearings to
criticize the criteria as well.

The boards in turn would criticize for Congress the
budgetary proposals and awards of the National Institutes
of Health and other federal health care research agencies.

These critiques would link research opportunities to the delivery system's operational needs.

A designated federal agency would provide staff support for the boards and would prepare analyses of the cost, manpower, and utilization requirements for major pieces of new medical equipment. Only limited numbers of hospitals would be permitted to use new equipment until accurate cost and efficacy data would be assembled.

Hospitals would be classified by type according to their ability to provide certain ranges of services. In order to avoid duplication of expensive equipment and services, hospitals would have to extent staff privileges to all physicians licensed by the state in which they provide care. Peer review panels would be required to sanction the continued access to limited distributed equipment and services of physicians based on their performance. With this arrangement there would be increased opportunity for the regionalization of certain medical procedures as the health services research literature indicates is preferable in terms of patient outcomes.[12]

The local planning agencies could continue to function, but their attention would focus on such tasks as lobbying for their areas before the boards and Congress, helping applicants to prepare appropriate proposals, and commenting on the suitability of applicants to meet local needs. Thus, they would be at last freed from their current dilemma of serving two masters.

The reforms proposed are intended to balance the relevant societal interests by providing an opportunity for the expression of cost containment interests as well as for the expression of access and quality of care interests. They do not seek to remove health investments from politics. Congress would have the political task of allocating capital resources to and within the health care sector. It would do so with the knowledge both of the pressure increases in health care expenditures placed on other governmental activities and of the desires of the public for improvements in health care services. The specific allocations would be made by boards controlled by those who pay for health services subject to consumer and professional appeals to Congress for review. The boards' obvious interest in cost control thus would have to be tempered by a sensitivity to access and quality interests. Appropriately, the outcome of these decision-making processes would not be predetermined, but rather would be left to the play of real political interests.

Democratic government, if it is to survive, must tame the appetites as well as the passions of the people. To say that reform is not possible is to ignore our own history. Much change has occurred in the delivery of health services in just the past two decades. As the providers of health care know, more is certain to come.

NOTES

1. The National Health Planning and Resource Development Act of 1974, like most other pieces of major legislation, had complex origins. Clearly the arrangements selected in the act for the planning of health care facilities were greatly influenced by traditional doctrines of federalism and by the structure of the then existing health care planning system. But given that the summer of 1974 was the culmination of the Watergate crisis, it is just as obvious that major steps in public policy, such as were embodied in the act, were not then being subject to the usual degree of congressional and executive scrutiny. For a detailed examination of the origins of the act, see the papers by Brown, Checkoway, and Raab in this volume.

2. For a discussion of the growth of experience rating in health insurance, see John Krizay and Andrew Wilson, *The Patient As Consumer: Health Care Financing in the United States* (Lexington, Mass.: Lexington Books, 1974), pp. 39-43; and Paul J. Feldstein, *Health Care Economics* (New York: John Wiley & Sons, 1979), pp. 138-141. The common practice is to use experience rating for group policies covering 100 or more members. Note Richard Ostuw and John S. Fry, "Funding of Employee Benefits," *Topics in Health Care Financing,* Vol. 6, No. 3 (Spring 1980), pp. 35-50. Although only 46 percent of private health insurance plans involved groups of over 100 in 1974, these plans accounted for 95 percent of covered workers for that year. See Table No. 552, *Statistical Abstract of the United States* (Washington, D.C.: Government Printing Office, 1979), p. 343.

3. For an elaboration of these points, see Drew Altman, Richard Greene, and Harvey M. Sapolsky, *Health Regulation and Planning: The New England Experience* (Ann Arbor, Mich.: Health Administration Press, forthcoming).

4. There are some exceptions. In Rochester, New York, most of the major employers use Blue Cross as their health care insurer and rely on a community rated plan. In Rhode Island, the state government negotiates hospital rate increases in cooperation with Blue Cross, which holds a substantial share of the private health insurance market.

5. P.L. 95-142 is intended to prevent state Medicaid programs from using late payments as a mechanism to reduce outlays.

6. Judgments gleaned from interviews with major employers in the Minneapolis/St. Paul area. These interviews are part of a larger study of employers' attitudes toward rising health care costs that I have conducted under a grant from the National Center for Health Services Research.

7. Too little has been written about the proprietary chains. A recent commentary on one firm is Gwen Kinhead, "Humana's Hard-Sell Hospitals," *Fortune* (November 17, 1980), pp. 68-81. Note also John A. Hill, "Inducements and Impediments for Private Corporate Investment in the Delivery of Health Services," in G. K. MacLeod and M. Perlman, Editors, *Health Care Capital: Competition and Control* (Cambridge, Mass.: Ballinger, 1978), pp. 193-224.

8. R. W. Rhein, Jr., "Health Lobbyists: Clout in the Corridors of Power," *Medical World News* (June 12, 1978), pp. 66-81.

9. On the structure of the biomedical research and education system, note the following: Stephen Strickland, *Science and Dread Disease* (Cambridge, Mass.: Harvard University Press, 1972); Stephen Strickland, *Research and the Health of Americans* (Lexington, Mass.: Lexington Books, 1978); Selma J. Mushkin, *Biomedical Research; Costs and Benefits* (Cambridge, Mass.: Ballinger, 1979); and National Academy of Sciences, *Medical Technology and the Health Care System* (Washington, D.C.: National Academy of Sciences, 1979).

10. Harvey M. Sapolsky, "Here Comes the Artificial Heart," *The Sciences*, Vol. 18, No. 10 (December 1978), pp. 25-28. See also "Government and the Development of the Artificial Heart," in Artificial Heart Assessment Panel, *The Totally Implantable Artificial Heart* (Bethesda, Md.: National Heart and Lung Institute, 1973), Appendix A.

11. Attempts to control medical technology are in their nascent form, absorbed as they are in debates over the appropriate methodologies to employ. The pressures to do

more, however, are growing. See John K. Iglehart, "The Cost and Regulation of Medical Technology's Future Policy Directions," *Health and Society* (Winter 1977), pp. 61-79; and Louise B. Russell, *Technology in Hospitals: Medical Advances and Their Diffusion* (Washington, D.C.: Brookings Institution, 1979).

12. Note especially, Harold S. Luft, John P. Bunker, and Alain C. Enthoven, "Should Operations Be Regionalized? An Empirical Study of the Relation Between Surgical Volume and Mortality," *New England Journal of Medicine,* Vol. 301, No. 25 (December 20, 1979), pp. 1364-1369; and Harold S. Luft, "The Relation Between Surgical Volume and Mortality: An Exploration of Causal Factors and Alternative Models," *Medical Care,* Vol. 18, No. 9 (September 1980), pp. 940-959.

CONSUMERISM IN HEALTH
PLANNING AGENCIES*

Barry Checkoway

*The Health Planning Resources Development Act of
1974 specified that governing boards of planning
agencies have a majority of consumer members.
The influence of these consumers has frequently
been weak compared to the influence of health care
provider board members. The 1979 amendments to the
health planning law incorporated moves to strengthen
the position of consumers in planning, responding
to concerns, voiced by many, that the intent of
the original law has not been realized. In this
paper, Checkoway describes and analyzes the methods
used by three HSAs to successfully incorporate the
consumer voice into health planning.*

INTRODUCTION

P.L. 93-641, the National Health Planning and Resources
Development Act of 1974, created a national network of
Health Systems Agencies (HSAs) with an emphasis on consumer participation in planning. Consumer majorities
were required by law in each HSA governing board. These
consumers were to be "broadly representative of the social,
economic, linguistic, and racial populations, geographic

---

*Earlier versions of selected paragraphs of this paper
have appeared in Checkoway (1979) and Checkoway (1980).

areas of the health service area, and major purchasers of health care," and were deemed "essential to the effective performance of an agency's function" (*Federal Register*, 1976). Consumer majorities in theory promised to be a strong force in determining the direction of local health care planning.

The act also provided an opportunity for health planning to "catch up" with the expanding participation movements of recent years (Langton, 1978). It provided for public notice and open meetings, for an opportunity to comment on agency plans, and for a public record of board proceedings (*Federal Register*, 1976). Subsequent agency functions prescribed by the federal government included provisions of public information and access to agency records and data, and made specific mention of such methods as newsletters, second-language translations, annual reports, subarea advisory councils, task forces, and public education programs (Bureau of Health Planning, 1977). Surely consumers stood to benefit from methods that would provide representation, improve communications, and activate participation.

In practice, however, the formation of health planning agencies has been no assurance of consumer active and effective participation. More than 200 HSAs have received federal designation, and in many cases consumers have had little real participation in planning. Most analyses of consumer participation under P.L. 93-641 have focused on the socially descriptive characteristics of consumer board members and other representational issues, with the general finding that consumer majorities are not always representative of their area population (Hyman, 1976; Clark, 1977; Orkand Corporation, 1977; Pastreich, 1977; Sypniewski and Semmel, 1977; Tannen, 1977; Marmor and Morone, 1980). Studies of participation practice itself have tended to find gaps between stated participation aims and actual practice (Consumer Commission on the Accreditation of Health Services, 1977; Knox, 1978; Paap, 1978; U.S. House Subcommittee on Health and the Environment, 1978; Kleiman, 1979; Checkoway, 1979). There are serious obstacles to the expansion of consumer participation in health planning. Some of these obstacles are administrative in nature, others relate to disparities in knowledge among the participants, yet others result from a lack of consumer constituency support and community organization.

Despite the obstacles, there are health planning agencies that have sought consumer participation with fervor. This does not suggest that these agencies are typical of the field, or that their methods might not be used elsewhere to frustrate and contain consumerism, or that independent consumer organization might not be a better way for some people to participate. It does suggest that there are agencies and methods that might be a source of practical ideas for those concerned about making consumer participation work. This paper describes three such agencies.

METHODOLOGY

This paper reports on a pilot study of HSAs which were judged to employ innovative methods to encourage consumer and community participation in health planning.* Innovative methods include those that facilitate the meaningful involvement of consumers and consumer organizations and are replicable elsewhere. Consumers are those participants who have no direct fiduciary interest in the outcomes of planning decisions.† The study sought to identify selected agencies, describe major methods, and analyze factors affecting participation.

Limited resources for this study constrained the research methodology and forced reliance on informed sources and a limited number of cases for analysis.†† In short, criteria were developed to evaluate agencies in relation

*This pilot study is based in part on research completed under contract to the Bureau of Health Planning and reported in Checkoway (1980). Subsequent research was undertaken through funding from the Office for Interdisciplinary Projects at the University of Illinois and the National Academy of Sciences.

† In this study, business and labor groups are not considered as consumers because of their fiduciary interest in health planning.

†† The research methodology is described more fully in Checkoway (1980).

to consumer participation; informed sources were asked to
nominate agencies according to the criteria; selected
agencies were asked to submit information on their methods;
site visits were arranged to gather information and materials; and interviews were conducted with individuals
at selected agencies and sites. Selection criteria were
derived from a search of major published, unpublished,
and draft HSA performance standards and guidelines and
from standard functional criteria employed in the participation field. Thirty informed sources, including federal
regional and headquarters health planning officials, HSA
board and staff members, local and national consumer leaders, and scholars and consultants concerned with health
planning were asked to nominate agencies. A short list
of agencies cited most frequently was developed. Site
visits were made to each selected agency to obtain information. Interviews were conducted with agency staff,
consumer and provider board members, and others. More
than 80 nonstandardized interviews were conducted, using
an interview schedule designed to guide questions related
to the research. The data were then evaluated, analyzed,
and prepared for presentation.

The findings reported here should be considered in
terms of the limitations of this approach. First, the
lack of comparative data on all agencies and methods makes
it difficult to conclude that those selected are the leading or only innovative agencies or methods in the field.
It is impossible to identify what is innovative or exem-
plary about a specific phenomenon without knowledge of
the overall field of which it is a part. Although the
major measure in the selection of agencies was their
reputation among highly informed sources, an expanded
cross-sectional national survey might identify other
agencies and methods.* Second, participation methods were
analyzed largely in terms of their scope, not in terms of
their impact on agency outputs or community systems. An
expanded study might assess and relate these outputs to
the quality of the methods themselves and the factors
affecting participation. Third, only a small number of
agencies could be studied. It is difficult to make broad

_____
*The author has undertaken such a survey in collaboration
with the Office for Interdisciplinary Projects and Survey
Research Laboratory at the University of Illinois.

judgments or draw general conclusions from a limited number of cases. An expanded study would allow more comprehensive analysis. Finally, these data present a snapshot of phenomena in a field that itself is in flux. The agencies studied might have changed in the interim. Despite its limitations, however, these data are still an available source of information on which to base preliminary conclusions and further research.

It can be reported at the outset that, despite the obstacles, there are health planning agencies that have undertaken consumer participation with fervor. Although each agency is unique, the overall range of methods is diverse and spans standard functional criteria employed in the participation field. In reviewing the variety of methods, some of the efforts are striking, as in the following cases not reported in depth:

1. An agency in a major metropolitan area on the West Coast has created and staffed six subarea advisory councils that operate like a federation of local governments. Community groups and neighborhood health centers have used the councils to press their own issues, including opposition to public hospital closures, investigations of nursing homes, and legislation for national health service physicians.

2. An agency that includes a large eastern industrial city has formed district area councils in addition to subarea advisory councils to facilitate participation at the neighborhood level. Consumer governing body members have formalized a consumer caucus that meets prior to meetings to exchange ideas, discuss agency items, and formulate strategies to represent their positions.

3. An agency covering a large rural area without a single central city applies a "coalitional planning" methodology to build support among community leaders and public officials who can affect planning. Agency staff conducted a power structure analysis to determine the community influentials and include them on agency board, subarea advisory councils, and committees (Mandel et al., 1980).

4. An agency in a large suburban area conducts public forums to inform and consult with consumers. Topics of forums include home health care, women's health, occupational health, and safety (Otto and Scott, 1980).

5. Another suburban agency provides technical assistance

and funding to groups forming community health councils
within subareas. These independent, grass roots councils
help identify local health problems and promote community
discussion of possible solutions. The agency provides
start-up funds; assistance in developing articles of
incorporation, bylaws, and media campaigns; and a regular
forum for meetings of health council representatives.
Twelve community health councils have formed, with expectations for formation of 10 more councils.

6. An agency in a major southern city employs a method
in which some consumer governing body members are selected
from and accountable to outside community groups. The
agency seeks to identify major groups and invites them to
participate in a caucus formed to select a representative
to the board. Local legal services and consumer advocacy
groups were instrumental in developing this method.

7. An agency in the rural Midwest helped develop a
Comprehensive School Health Education Program to assist
area school systems to formulate curricula and prepare
programs to educate students in grades K-12 about health
problems and alternatives for dealing with them (Wahlfeldt
and Wilkinson, 1980).

8. This same agency has created a plan development fund
to provide direct funding to independent community groups
proposing activities supportive of agency plans. A standing committee of the board invites and reviews proposals,
excluding providers and proposals to construct or modern-
ize medical facilities. The agency has funded a community
group proposing to educate senior citizens about fraudu-
lent insurance plans (Wahlfeldt and Wilkinson, 1980).

INNOVATIVE CONSUMERISM IN HEALTH PLANNING AGENCIES

This section describes three agencies that were ranked
highest for their efforts to encourage consumer participation in planning. The descriptions are designed to capture some of the elements of the innovative agencies and
methods and capture some of the factors affecting participation as a form of innovation in planning. The descriptions are to the extent possible taken directly from agency
site visits, interviews, and materials. The aim is to

describe each agency in the words of its principal participants and documents.*

West Bay Health Systems Agency

The West Bay is a culturally diverse urban area that
stretches the length of San Francisco along its western
shores. The main city of San Francisco has attracted a
diverse range of ethnic and cultural groups; suburban
Marin and San Mateo counties help expand this diversity.
Although health care resources are among the finest in
the world, an excess of hospitals has fueled a costly
technology race, and access to care remains a problem
for persons with language difficulties or unable to pay
(West Bay Health Systems Agency, 1979).
    The West Bay has a history of public participation and
consumer activism. Consumer leaders with technical knowledge and political skills are familiar figures before
local councils and committees. In some cases they have
sought representation and gained leadership positions on
these councils. Neighborhood associations and ethnic
groups have sprung up with vocal constituencies. In issues
such as neighborhood preservation and institutional expansion, they have formed powerful coalitions to exercise
influence and win rewards. The planning environment is
characterized by open competition in which community
groups play an active role (Jones, 1972; Hartman, 1974;
Wirt, 1974).
    It was logical that consumer activities would perceive
the HSA as a vehicle for participation. A West Bay HSA
Community Coalition intervened in the agency application
and designation process on behalf of affirmative action
principles and decentralization of planning through subarea advisory councils. Consumers on the initial governing body included activists representing civil rights and
neighborhood interests and seeking to increase access,

---

*Textual references to agency documents represent only
a sample of those employed. Direct quotations are from
site interviews unless otherwise noted.

eliminate language barriers, and challenge hospitals to meet local needs. Subsequent consumer representatives were instrumental in hiring an executive director who viewed the agency as a force for social change and who himself hired staff committed to this belief (Grant, 1980). The executive director today is described as an "activist" and "risk taker" on behalf of consumerism who is "willing to challenge the status quo."

Consumers participate largely through three subarea advisory councils. These councils establish committees, elect officers, deliberate on plan development and implementation, and select 27 of 30 governing body members (West Bay Health Systems Agency, 1978a). Consumer board members view these councils as a vehicle to address local health issues. Some of these consumers spend unusual amounts of time to "make sure that consumer viewpoints are expressed on every issue," "maintain close contact with community groups," and "build political alliances necessary to win key votes for consumers." One consumer leader describes the agency as "a public forum in which community groups might have equal footing with medical institutions," another as "a vehicle for community organizing in health care." These consumers are joined by selected provider board members, drawn from nonphysician occupational groups, who also express strong consumer viewpoints.

Three staff professionals serve as county coordinators to assist the subarea advisory councils in facilitating participation. They recruit members from diverse community groups, assure compliance with federal representational requirements, and advocate for low-income and minority consumers. One coordinator described efforts to "open up the health political process," another to "give people the feeling that they can control the decisions affecting their lives." Special efforts were made to recruit coordinators from among key minority groups and with special skills in advocacy planning and community organization. One previously served as an advocacy planner, another as leader of a major health consumer group, another as state-wide leader of Raza Alliance in HSAs. The agency assigns the coordinators full-time to this function, gives them high position in the agency, and pays them equivalent to senior planners (West Bay Health Systems Agency, 1978a).

The agency developed its first health systems plan by producing draft working papers that were formulated in community workshops, discussed by each subarea advisory council, and then circulated to more than 3,750 individuals and groups, including low-income, civil rights, and women's groups. Comments were received, incorporated in draft plans, discussed in public hearings in each subarea, and then revised, adopted, and approved (West Bay Health Systems Agency, 1978b; West Bay Health Systems Agency, 1979). The HSA recommendation to eliminate excess hospital beds, supported by agency data recommending closure of selected hospitals, has provided a health planning issue that is specific and deeply felt in the community.

The implementation and review mechanism itself resulted from consumer participation. In the mid-1970s, a neighborhood coalition formed to stop the planned expansion of two local hospitals and to propose a master plan ordinance that today gives the agency authority to conduct reviews, employ public hearings and other procedures allowing input, and requires hospitals to develop institutional master plans and make these plans public (San Francisco Municipal Code, 1976). Two highly significant reviews under this ordinance recommended denial of expansion projects, focused attention on the problem of excess capacity and the need for joint planning, and created a climate for change in the hospital industry. The president of the local medical society has called for closure of several hospitals and of more than a quarter of the city's beds.

A major vehicle for public information is the *West Bay Communique,* the agency's monthly newsletter. The *West Bay Communique* is sent to over 4,000 individuals and groups and includes extended, analytic articles from a strong consumer perspective. Among the issues covered are hospital mergers, excess hospital beds, multicultural health services, consumer rights, and health problems of specific groups. The newsletter has become the leading vehicle for health planning information in the area. The monthly tabloid presents an attractive appearance, makes liberal use of illustrations and cartoons, and is translated into Spanish and Chinese. The editor, who previously wrote a syndicated consumer column in newspapers throughout California, takes a consistent consumer orientation. The editorial orientation was questioned by local providers but defended by the governing body. Other agency public information activities include legal notices of hearings and meetings, public service announcements, radio and television appearances, mass mailings, leaflet distribution, slide presentations, multilingual plans, and personal outreach efforts.

The agency employs public forums to increase awareness of health planning issues. Following reports of difficult conditions at San Francisco General Hospital, a public hospital serving underserved groups and others, the agency sponsored a forum at the hospital. Agency staff notified key community groups, arranged speakers, and circulated flyers throughout the community. Many residents spoke out in support of the hospital and asked that constructive action be taken. Shortly thereafter, local elected officials asked the HSA to undertake a study of the factors affecting the future of the hospital. The completed report provided information for action in support of the hospital.

The agency has shown consistent commitment to affirmative action and minority participation. Agency staff place special emphasis on promoting the participation of those that are medically underserved or suffer the effects of discrimination. The agency conducted a special recruitment program to develop and maintain a workforce that mirrors the demographic characteristics of the area. Consultants, themselves drawn from ethnic minorities in the health field, were retained to recruit staff from among those with known interest in expanding employment opportunities for minorities, including civil rights and low-income advocacy groups. A recent study of HSA representation and parity identified the agency board and staff as the most racially integrated in the state and as an example for others to follow.

In efforts to involve ethnic minorities and medically underserved people, two recent developments merit special description. First, Latino governing body members have formed La Raza Health Alliance to unite Raza health organizations and provide a basis for advocacy on behalf of Latinos in health planning. They requested one county coordinator to initiate La Raza HSA to bring together Latino consumers to discuss common concerns, review meeting agendas, and develop action strategies. Second, minority consumers have initiated a Task Force on Language Access to Health Care to address issues of particular concern to minorities. Among present task force activities is a survey of local hospitals, clinics, and other health facilities to assess bilingual health care services and develop strategies for improvement.

Overall, in a culturally diverse urban area with a history of participation, consumer activists have perceived the HSA as a vehicle for community organization, sought representation and leadership positions, and worked to influence agency development. It is not surprising

that the HSA appears as an advocacy agency on behalf of
vigorous participation, affirmative action, and minority
representation.

Health Systems Agency of Northern Virginia

Northern Virginia, located in the suburbs of Washington,
D.C., is not an average American community. It is among
the most affluent areas in Virginia and one of the wealth-
iest in the nation (Health Systems Agency of Northern
Virginia, 1979a). Many residents are employed by government and recognize the value of government intervention
and overall planning. The Washington metropolitan area
has a tradition of regional planning that includes regional
planning bodies, councils of government, and aggregations
of counties joined through joint powers agreements. These
bodies tend to operate as representative councils in which
public officials or their representatives make decisions
on behalf of their constituents.

The HSA is organized as part of a nonprofit corporation
sponsored by local governmental units and the regional
planning body. The agency apportions representatives
according to the population size of each jurisdiction and
specifies the qualifications needed to produce a representative board. Consumer board members mirror the area population and thus rank higher than the national average in
their income, education, and occupational status. One
consumer board member characterized her counterparts as
highly educated individuals using the HSA as a vehicle to
apply specialized interests and analytic skills to regional
health problems. She described consumers as able to analyze
highly technical information, take strong positions, and
express themselves with authority. The 30-member board
of directors are appointed from and accountable to public
elected officials and regional planning commissioners,
who themselves may be accepted or rejected in periodic
elections. Like its local counterparts, the HSA thus
operates as a council of representatives. The approach
is one in which the agency keeps the public informed
while representatives make decisions.

The agency places emphasis on methods to inform and
consult with the public. These information provision
methods include legal notices of hearings and meetings,
news releases and public service announcements, newsletters,
direct mass mail, and public presentations. For example,

a speaker's bureau facilitates board and staff member presentations before local service clubs and civic groups. Although the principal function is to provide information, the bureau also allows agency representatives to exchange ideas and receive feedback; enhances board-staff relations through collaboration for presentations; and serves as a form of board member education and leadership training. Prospective speakers generally must update their knowledge, sharpen their understanding, and learn to act as spokesmen for health planning. It is no surprise that the bureau has operated as a training ground for agency leadership.

The agency has published the most detailed physicians' directory in the nation (Health Systems Agency of Northern Virginia, 1979b). The directory provides basic information about local hospitals, health departments, and health maintenance organizations in addition to physician backgrounds, practices, and fees. The directory also indicates whether physicians speak foreign languages, serve patients with special problems, and equip their offices for the handicapped. Approximately 5,000 copies of the directory are distributed free of charge at a production cost of roughly $20,000. To complete the directory, the agency was forced to challenge the constitutionality of a state law prohibiting physicians from providing information about their practices and to confront opposition from local medical society representatives who used the media to criticize the HSA project. In addition to this project, this agency has published a consumer guide to nursing homes with information about charges, services, alternatives to nursing home care, and available financial assistance (Health Systems Agency of Northern Virginia, 1979c).

The HSA has taken strong public positions on health issues and included these positions in agency plans. The annual implementation plan originally included positions on abortion rights and gun controls, stating first that low-income persons should not be denied any family planning services, including abortion services, because of inability to pay, and later that the public health would be better protected if guns were controlled and used properly. The agency then wrote letters to congressmen and state legislators on behalf of these positions. In response, representatives of the county medical society, private physicians and dentists, and antiabortion groups protested the use of public funds to advocate such positions. Right-to-Life members attended HSA board meetings and employed

drilled into them just in case one of the dead happened
to be alive. This was expensive, but it was worth the
trouble. A second group came up with an inexpensive and
more efficient idea. Each coffin would have a 12-inch
stake affixed to the inside of the coffin lid, exactly
at the level of the heart. When the coffin was closed,
all uncertainty would cease.

There is no record as to the solution chosen by the
people of Lithuania--but for our purposes here, the important consideration is that the two different solutions
were generated by two different questions about the same
problem. The first solution was an answer to the question:
"How can we make sure that we do not bury people who are
still alive?" The second was an answer to the question:
"How can we make sure that everyone we bury is dead?"[7]

As long as the planning mystique prevails, consumers
will fail to look for the policies inherent in the planning propositions (agendas) presented them. Without clear
awareness of these propositions, there is no way consumers
can move to bend planning policy in the direction of their
own priorities and concerns. Until the consumer questions
the planning agenda itself (whether the ultimate outcomes
be affirmation or negation), the consumer cannot take
charge of the process, cannot effectuate strategies directed toward his or her own goals. The agenda is out of
control (consumer control). The consumer has been high-
jacked, if you will, undertaking a journey toward a destina-
tion that may, or may not, be in his or her desired direction.

Just as the concept of health planning as technology
masks the political process that is health planning, so it
suppresses effective consumer action by distorting perception of appropriate action. In December 1979, Health
Resources Administration officials issued the following
statement to the National Health Planning Council, which
was then studying potential consumer priorities: "To
what extent does the Council want the health planning
process to become an advocacy system for specific categorical segments of the underserved, and how do you reconcile
this type of approach in a planning system that is directed
at broad service delivery systems improvement and cost
containment? There seem to be conflicting philosophies
and roles being promoted by the Council and by other forces
in the health planning program."

Here, it seems to me, we have the consumer agenda
framed as "an advocacy system for specific categorical

elements of the´ underserved." Mystification takes many
forms indeed. Here we have yet another attempt to maintain that consumers should not *have* an agenda (at least,
not in the planning process)--and to imply that *other*
interests are neutral (represent the broad public interest).
It is a tactic that presents an almost impossible dilemma
to consumer representatives. Consumers definitively represent specific constituencies, specific perspectives,
and specific experiential expertise (at least, they do
if they have been selected through an accountable process).
*Their competency resides in their ability to voice the
point of view of their particular constituency.* Yet,
would they do so, they are often told they "have an ax
to grind," "represent a limited interest," or "reflect
a special population only." Assertion of specific needs
is advocacy, and, in my view, competent and effective
advocacy for special populations (are not they all?) is
both an input to and an outcome of competent public
interest planning. I believe consumers have succeeded
so poorly in seizing agenda control in part because they
have tried so little. There has been so little effort
primarily because consumers bought the notion that planning is a technical process. Needed is affirmation that
no one in health planning represents other than a "point
of view" (and that includes planners); that no one represents the "broad public interest"; no one is neutral; and
that everyone is involved in advocacy--whether subtlely,
through control of the agenda by quiet, in-house administrative processes, or through full-scale public debate.
Clarity regarding these few notions could go a long way to
giving back to the consumer the strength of his or her
own motive power.

What we have now, then, is the mystification of the
politics of health. We call this process health planning.
As usual, technicalization serves its purpose. The American Medical Association has frequently been accused--by
both consumers and planners--of mystification of the process of health. The phenomenon is no different in health
planning. I doubt that the motives are different. I am
sure that the outcomes are not.

ENABLING CONSUMER CONTROL

Unity

We have talked of the need for consumer control and of the impact of loss of control on consumer effectiveness. What must occur to enable consumers to take control?

It is axiomatic that the consumer movement cannot be effective if it is divided. The array of consumer interests must build an agenda, a platform, about which a broad constituency shares enthusiasm, or consumers will never be able to compete with vested interests. Quite simply, it is imperative to the consumer movement that the philosophical framework for alliance and action be affirmation of the right of every person to the level and type of health care he or she needs, at whatever age, in whatever condition. Choice for or against health interventions must ultimately reside with the individual involved, be that intervention preventive maintenance for the well, or secondary or tertiary intervention for the ill. Consumer coalitions must center on the conviction that this nation can afford the health care its consumers choose. The definition of affordable is primarily determined by valuation. If there is to be a strong consumer movement, there is no alternative organizing framework, for within the context in which any life is deemed expendable, the potential for coalition dissolves. It is so easy to play families confronted with the anguish of birth defects and developmental disabilities against the needs of the underserved minority populations; the desires of the victims of leukemia against the interests of those deprived of the most primary of care. The consumer movement cannot afford to entertain these kinds of trade-offs. *Whatever cost savings are to be achieved must come from reduction in waste, improved productivity, prevention of unnecessary illness, not in diversion of needed resources from one population to another, and not in targeting one population or another as nondeserving of health care assistance.*

Planning Based on Consumer Perceived Need

Consumer control implies responsiveness to consumer needs. Often, services inventory approaches to planning are substituted for needs assessment. Providers say, "Let us

investigate the adequacy of our current services in relationship to their availability throughout the community,
then we will know what service duplication exists and
what service gaps there are, and we can work to fill those
gaps so that we have a more comprehensive service delivery
system." Essentially, that is how the planning agencies
work now. The primary task is to determine, on the basis
of federal formulas, whether a community has too much
or too little of a particular type of service. Such an
agenda may seem reasonable. It is, however, quite simply
a way of saying, "Let us find out where we can deliver more
of the kinds of services we are delivering now." It is
a status quo, business-as-usual mentality. The questions
seldom asked of clients or consumers are: "What are your
needs? What kind of governmental response is the most
appropriate response, or is a change in community living
conditions, legislation, or regulation more likely to
produce desired outcomes? Or is a combination of services
and reforms needed?

Most planning is undertaken on the basis of perceptions
and data supplied by service providers, and not on the
basis of assessed desires of current and prospective
clients of services. In most planning activities, the
perceptions of citizens and consumers are ignored or inun-
dated by service statistics for current or projected
interventions.[8] Yet, the interests and needs of service
providers and those of consumers are often very different.
Needs data is the baseline for consumer-oriented planning.
Only when planning discussions proceed on the basis of
citizen-perceived needs do consumers have a handle on
policy formulation--a chance to direct planning policy toward effective responses to their priority needs. If
planning is isolated from systematic assessment of citizen-
perceived need, there is no possibility for citizen impact.
The ball is irretrievably in the provider court.

In consumer-needs-based planning, the focus is on the
outcome desired by the citizen. Once a desired outcome
is known, it is possible to structure responses, and to
structure them in the most cost-efficient manner compatible
with the desired outcome, but the focus never leaves the
problems of the citizens.

What, then, would a consumer-oriented, needs-based
planning model look like?

1. It would begin with the citizen in the policy role,
setting priorities regarding services citizens want and
for which they are willing to pay.

221

2. It would assure that the full array of consumer perspectives are fully involved in planning. Instead of setting up shop, providing public notice, and declaring it the
"responsibility of consumers to come to us," planning would
seek out the consumer most at risk--the consumer without
political experience and skills, the consumer with transportation problems, the chronically ill and the homebound,
the consumer undergoing serious health care interventions,
families of the long-term seriously ill or terminally ill,
consumers of trauma resources, ethnic minorities with language and cultural differences, the deaf and blind with
their special communications problems, the handicapped, and
children--who are spoken for only if someone happens to
remember. . . . Without special outreach, health planning
omits those populations most at risk, and the rich experience of people who know human need in the health care
sphere first hand, by living its problems and challenges--
is lost to the planning process.

3. It would rely heavily on citizen perception of need,
and on analysis of context, community conditions, community priorities, and desired outcomes.

4. *The HSA would have the authority and the funds to re-
ward providers desiring to implement coordinated consumer
responsive systems of care identified as needed in health
planning activities.* Failure to provide HSAs this capacity
can be fatal to any attempt to achieve either effective
consumer policymaking or important health systems changes.

5. It would involve citizens in evaluation of funded
programs, measured against clearly stated performance
standards, and would provide policymakers ample opportunity
to rethink periodically their funding decisions and to re-
cycle the design process to take advantage of lessons
wrought by experience.

MEASURES OF CONSUMER RESPONSIVENESS

Given the exploration we have made, what are the measures
by which we might assess the likelihood that any planning
model would encourage (or allow) consumer effectiveness?
Let us consider measures in relation to the dynamics that
I have maintained effect consumer control:

A. *Control and Role*
   --extent to which consumers set policy (as opposed
to administering the policy of others)

--degree to which consumers own (as opposed to the
degree to which whey share or are excluded from) the controlling positions in health planning
   --degree to which planning is affirmed as a political activity and extent to which consumers are provided
training about planning as a political process as opposed
to training in technology of planning
   --degree to which planning is affirmed as a form
of advocacy
   --degree to which staff of health planning agencies
is accountable to consumers, i.e., hired and fired by consumers, and accountable solely to consumers (as opposed to
shared with vested interests)

   B. *Agenda-Setting*
   --degree to which consumers determine planning
agendas (as opposed to sharing the development of agendas
with vested interests)
   --degree to which planning activities reflect the
purpose of consumers

   C. *Language*
   --degree to which the language of the planning
agendas and outcome documents is the language of consumers
   --degree to which planning jargon coincides with
the word choices, values, policies, and purposes of consumers

   D. *Alliance*
   --degree to which planning allows consumers to
work together to achieve consumer goals and priorities instead of working against each other to "win" for a specific
target group

   E. *Planning Approach*
   --degree to which planning approaches are needs-
based, emphasizing citizen-perceived need, the context in
which interventions and desired outcomes are offered

   F. *Planning Approach and Prerogatives*
   --degree to which staff have the skills to clearly
identify and develop policy options supportive of consumer
agendas
   --extent to which outreach is provided to the full
array of consumers, and the degree to which consumers are
assisted in formulating their concerns, are assisted in
carrying these concerns forward consistently within the

planning process, and extent to which outcomes are accountable to consumers
  --degree to which the planning system promotes
evaluation of process toward desired goals
  --degree to which the planning system integrates
funding policy and reimbursement guarantees for consumers
and providers attempting health care arrangements compatible with health systems plans

SUMMARY

Clearly, planning model options are numerous. The inter-
play of role definitions, expectations, accountability,
control of agenda, language, philosophical frameworks,
and methodology in any given model can, in varying combinations, produce innumerable variations in outcomes. But
the most significant choice from a consumer perspective is
the choice we make regarding the *role* of the citizen-consumer in health planning.
  In short, we can accept the concept of planning as a
function of the provider industry, with consumers invited
to make input in the provider house.
  We can accept the concept of planning as a form of
syndicalism, with the array of vested interests negotiating the division of health care allocations, and consumers' participation merely one input among the array of
vested interests.
  We can accept a model in which the third-party payors--
public and private--are hosts and directors of the process
through which health care resources, which fiscal inter-
mediaries consider scarce, are divided.
  Or we can insist on "public interest" planning, in
which citizens determine what they are willing to afford,
hire, and direct planning staff to assist in designing
optimal strategies for implementation of consumer policies
and invite providers to negotiate the terms under which
strategies will be carried out.
  Each model is, of course, available, but all but the
last sets the stage for citizen-consumer co-optation.

REFERENCES

1. Institute of Medicine. *Health Planning in the*
United States: Issues in Guideline Development.

(Washington, D.C.: National Academy of Sciences, March 1980), p. 8.

2. *Ibid.*, p. 10.

3. *Ibid.*, p. 27.

4. *Ibid.*, p. 10.

5. U.S. Congress, Senate, Committee on Governmental Affiars. *Prepaid Health Plans and Health Maintenance Organizations.* Report No. 95-749 (U.S. Government Printing Office, Washington, D.C., 1978).

6. Health Resources Administration, Health and Human Services. "Involvement of Chronically Ill and Disabled Populations in the Planning Process."

7. Postman, Neil. *Crazy Talk, Stupid Talk* (New York: Garden City Press, 1974).

8. Strauss, M. B., and C. B. Vance. *Indicators in Social Planning* (Yale University Press, October 1970), p. 152.

MODELS OF REPRESENTATION:
CONSUMERS AND THE HSAs*

James A. Morone

*Almost no provision of P.L. 93-641 has engendered
as much confusion and discussion as the requirements
for consumer representation on the governing boards
of health planning agencies. In this paper Morone
presents the theoretical bases of public participation in policy making. He relates the language
of P.L. 93-641 and subsequent amendments to the
theoretical bases, and describes the political,
legal, and administrative problems that occurred.
Some suggestions for overcoming such problems are
offered.*

PREFACE

The National Health Planning and Resources Development Act
authorized a national network of local health planning

---

* I wish to thank Theodore Marmor for his extraordinary--
always challenging--assistance. Marmor coauthored an
early version of this article, which appeared in the
Health Law Project Library Bulletin (April 1979). We have
also published considerably different versions of these
topics in *Health and Society* (Winter 1980) and *Ethics*
(forthcoming, Spring 1981). The topics discussed here
are more fully dealt with in part of my forthcoming
dissertation on "Consumer Representation, Public Planning
and Democratic Theory."

agencies. Over 200 Health Systems Agencies (HSAs) were
to be numerically dominated by health care consumers
(51 to 60 percent of each governing board) working with
local providers (who formed the rest of the board) and a
professional staff.

Consumer representation accompanied an ambitious conception of health planning itself. The new program was to
produce "scientific planning with teeth," cut medical care
costs, improve access to medical care, and assure its high
quality. HSAs were to pursue these ambitious goals through
a mix of plan making and regulatory activities.

More than any element in the program, the effort to
empower consumers triggered confusion and controversy.
The original legislation (P.L. 93-641) was quickly mired in
the effort to institute consumer representation. Three
years later, amendments to the Health Planning Act (P.L.
96-79) vitiated some major difficulties, ignored others,
and simply passed some through to the local HSAs.

This paper's aim is to untangle the theoretical and political difficulties that have snared the law's effort to
enhance consumer representation. I try to lay out a "conceptual map" of representation and related concepts; both
the original legislation and its subsequent amendments
are fixed in relation to them. Stated broadly, the focus
of this paper is on the theoretical, legal, and administrative questions raised by the efforts to create boards
governed by consumers who are "broadly representative" of
local constituents.

EARLY DIFFICULTIES

P.L. 93-641 was plain enough about consumer majorities on
HSAs. The statute required between 51 and 60 percent of
every board to be consumers, "broadly representative of
the social, economic, linguistic, and racial populations
. . . of the area."[1] But the law and its regulations were
silent on the details of implementing this mandate. How
representatives were to be chosen, for instance, was
ignored. Which demographic groups should dominate under
the broad headings of social, linguistic, and economic
representation was not addressed. The clearest representational requirement was that metropolitan and nonmetropolitan representatives precisely mirror their proportions
in the population at large.

Disputes over consumer roles in health planning reached the courts almost immediately, exposing the conceptual difficulties of the law's model of representation. Several suits claimed inadequate means for selecting consumer representatives. But a New York court ruled in *Aldamuy* v. *Pirro* that there were no criteria by which it could choose between two competing minority representatives even if one had been selected by election.[2] As long as the requisite *number* of a particular minority were board members, the law's representation requirements were satisfied. A district court in Texas determined that requisite number by referring to the census tract.[3]

In *Rakestraw* v. *Califano* and other cases, various social groups sued demanding seats on the local board; the law and its regulations incorporated no principles for differentiating those with valid objections from those with merely frivolous ones.[4] Across the nation, HSAs scrambled to find poor, even uneducated consumers in a legally mandated, but conceptually misguided, effort to mirror the demographic characteristics of their area. And after selection, the problems of effective consumer representation continued to bedevil the HSA boards. Many members—chosen merely for their descriptive qualities (e.g., income level, race)—had no idea whom they spoke for and, in places, were unwilling to attend meetings.

In short, administrators quickly discovered that achieving meaningful consumer representation requires considerably more than simply calling for it in a law. Rather, it requires some fundamental theoretical choices. Decisions must be made about the selection of representatives, what those representatives should be like, and the expectations that should govern their behavior.

Whom the representatives are to represent—the constituencies—is also a puzzle when geographic representation is supplemented or abandoned. In addition, the organizational structures within which the representatives operate must be specified. Do they enhance or impede effective representation? Is the tendency toward imbalanced political markets (and in this case the domination of health care providers) redressed?

These questions cannot be avoided. The success of consumer representation is contingent on how they get answered. Many of the early failures of P.L. 93-641 follow from a failure to even consider them directly.

CONCEPTUAL PUZZLES: ACCOUNTABILITY AND PARTICIPATION

There are three topics central to consumer involvement in
P.L. 93-641 that have been conceptually muddled, both in
the law itself and in the analysis and litigation surrounding it. They are accountability, participation, and representation.

Accountability

Put simply, accountability means "answering to"--or more
precisely--"having to answer to." One must answer to agents
who control scarce resources one desires. In the classic
electoral example, officials are accountable to voters because they control the scarce resource officials desire.
Public officials are accountable to legislatures that control funds, pressure groups who can extend or withdraw
support, or even medical providers who can choose whether
to cooperate with an official's program.
  The crucial element in each case is that accountability
stems from some resource valued by the accountable actor.
Accountability is thus not merely an ideal, like honesty,
which public actors "ought" to strive toward. Rather, the
disposition of valued scarce resources will hang in the
balance, manipulated by the relevant constituency.
  I call the means by which actors are held to account
"mechanisms of accountability." These mechanisms can vary
enormously in character and in the extent of control they
impose. For example, voters can occasionally exert some
control with a "yes" or "no" decision, whereas work supervisors can regularly monitor a subordinate's work, enforcing
compliance with specific demands.
  There is often, to be sure, a give-and-take process in
which actors try to maximize their freedom of action and
thus minimize accountability. And those indifferent to the
scarce resources in question (e.g., an official with no desire to be reelected) are not, strictly speaking, accountable. But this illustrates the crucial point: in speaking
of accountability, one must be able to point to specific
scarce resources--a particular mechanism--holding representatives to account.
  Many of the HSA requirements that are touted as enhancing accountability to the public are, in fact, irrelevant
to it:

- a public record of board proceedings;[5]
- open meetings, with the notice of meetings published in two newspapers and an address given where a proposed agenda may be obtained;[6]
- an opportunity to comment, either in writing, or in a public meeting, about designation,[7] or Health Systems Plans (HSPs),[8] or Annual Implementation Plans (AIPs).[9]

These requirements might be said to facilitate public accounting, not accountability. Public participation and information can inform the exercise of accountability, but without formal mechanisms forcing boards to answer to consumers, there is no direct public accountability.

Well-defined mechanisms of accountability are central to a strong conception of accountability. Propositions that substitute notions like "winning over" or "working with" the community for an identifiable mechanism are much weaker, conflating one common language usage of accounting for action with the stronger view of accountability to a constituency.

Suggesting that HSA agencies would be ineffective without public support is an equally weak conception of accountability to consumers. Every agency of government expresses these expectations and fears. What is unique about representative government is that the citizenry, not government agencies, is given the final "say." And the "say" of the citizenry is not expressed by "inhospitality" or "lack of trust" or "written protests" but by an authoritative decision institutionalized as a mechanism of accountability.

Accountability can be to more than one constituency. As health planning was originally cast, DHHS, state government, local government, consumers, providers, and numerous other groups could all attempt to hold an HSA to account. These competing agents can introduce considerable tension. The most long-standing conflict lies between accountability to local and to national government. Both conceptions are rooted in classic traditions of democratic theory.[10]

The emphasis on community control rests on utilitarian and Jeffersonian traditions and has been seized upon by opponents of big government and centralized bureaucracies. Local communities, according to this view, best understand their own needs and ought, therefore, to be responsible for the policies by which they are governed.

The opposing position draws from sources as disparate as Marx and Weber, Madison, and Hamilton. National needs require national solutions. What is good for individual

communities (e.g., the best hospitals) may not sum to what
is best for the entire nation (lower medical costs). This
conception typically expresses egalitarian values--only a
national policy can redistribute costs and benefits among
states and regions.

Since the operating rules of each HSA were to be established locally, the potential for local accountability was
present. However, insofar as the law took up the issue
explicitly, it pressed accountability to HEW (significantly,
only 5 HSAs are units of local government).

HEW is responsible for reviewing the plans, structure
and operation of every agency at least once every 12
months.[11] Renewal of designation, and funding, is annually
at stake. This is accountability in every important sense.
But it can be traced to the public only by the long theoretical strand leading through the presidency. From this
perspective, HSA boards are no more accountable to the
public than any other federal executive agency, certainly
a far cry from the rhetoric than accompanied P.L. 93-641's
enactment.

The planning amendments facilitate a shifting in the
accountability of board members (if not the entire Health
Systems Agencies). The amendments limit "self selection"--
the choosing of new governing board representatives by the
HSA itself--to one-half of the board. HSAs are left to
devise their own process for selecting (at least) the other
half. In effect, the law requires that half the governing
board members be accountable to some element in the community. In any case, the accountability to local constituencies, so prominent in the rhetoric of P.L. 93-641, first
appears--tentatively, indirectly--in the amendments, P.L.
96-79.

Participation

In classical political thought, self-government meant direct
citizen participation in public decisions. In this context,
Plato envisioned a republic small enough for an orator to
address; Aristotle, one in which each citizen could know
every other. Rousseau argued that democracy ended when
participation did. Such conditions are largely absent in
modern industrial societies, making direct participation
largely anachronistic. Representation has come to replace
direct participation as the institutionalization of the
idea that "every man has the right to have a say in what
happens to him."[12]

The rhetoric of the 1974 planning law emphasized consumer representation.* The law itself, by contrast, concentrated on guidelines for direct public participation. Direct participation provisions tend to reinforce the political dominance of medical providers over consumers. Hospital administrators, state medical association officials, and other employed medical personnel are far more likely to pay the costs of participating in open HSA meetings, for their occupations are at issue. The general public is not likely to do so.

Furthermore, the difficulties of fostering direct consumer participation are aggravated by the nature of most health issues. Health concerns, though important, are intermittent for most people.[13] They are not as clearly or regularly salient as the condition of housing or children's schools--situations citizens confront daily. It is far more difficult to establish public participation in HSAs than in renter's associations or school districts.[14]

The point is not that participation is objectionable or that it should be stricken from the planning act; rather, without being tied to accountability and the representation of consumer health interests, the provisions for participation are of marginal use to consumers. They are more likely to be utilized by aroused provider institutions.

The new amendments did not, significantly, alter this balance (excepting the provision referred to in the preceding section and two highly circumscribed instances where meetings may be closed).[15] Nevertheless, much debate and rhetoric and advocacy continue to surround the participatory impulses of the planning act. They are surely destined to disappoint. Participatory provisions, central to an acceptable substitute for representative government, fail to make the crucial connection between intermittently vocalizing consumer concerns and institutionalizing representation in

---

*After the law was passed, there was a proliferation of brochures and pamphlets urging participation and promising accountability to local constituents. Academic commentary used similar language. As just one example, see Wayne Clark, "Placebo and Cure, State and Local Health Planning Agencies in the South," Southern Governmental Monitoring Project, Southern Regional Council, Atlanta, 1977, pp. 11-12.

an ongoing fashion. This type of participation may be a
necessary condition for effective consumer representation
and accountability. However, without being tied to mechanisms of accountability and a broad view of representation,
it is at best marginally useful to consumers.

REPRESENTATION

Representation is necessitated by the limits imposed on
direct, participatory democracy in modern society. The entire population cannot be present to make decisions. Hence,
institutions must be designed to "represent"--literally
"to make present again" or to "make present in some sense
something which is nevertheless not present literally or
in fact."[16]

Three aspects of representation are usually considered
in the appraisal of representative institutions: descriptive, substantive, and formal features.[17]

Descriptive Representation

Descriptive representation, the type of representation originally embedded in P.L. 93-641, emphasizes the characteristics of representatives. Since constituencies cannot be
present themselves to make public choices, the descriptive
model calls for a representative "body which [is] an exact
portrait, in miniature, of the people at large." The
argument is straightforward. Since all the people cannot
be present to make decisions, representative bodies ought
to be miniature versions--microcosms--of the public they
represent. The similarity of composition is expected to
result in similarity of outcomes; as John Adams put it, the
assembly will "think, feel, reason and [therefore] act" as
the public would have.[18]

A number of difficulties make this formulation problematic. First, "the public" is a broad category. What aspect
of it ought to be reflected in a representative body?

John Stuart Mill argued that opinions should be represented; Bentham and James Mill emphasized subjective
interests; Sterne, a more ambiguous "opinions, aspirations
and wishes"; Burke, broad fixed interest. Swabey suggested
that citizens were equivalent units, that if all had roughly
equal political opportunities, representatives would be a
proper random selection, and, consequently, descriptively

representative. Whichever the case, a failure to specify precisely what characteristics are represented reduces microcosm theories to incoherence.

Even when the relevant criteria for selecting representatives are properly specified, mirroring an entire nation is impossible. Mill's "every shade of opinion," for example, cannot be reconstructed in the assembly hall on one issue, much less on every. One cannot construct a microcosm of a million consumers no matter which 16, 17, or 18 consumers represent them on the HSA governing board. Competing opinions or interests can of course be represented. But the chief aim of microcosmic representation is mirroring the full spectrum of constituencies. Pitkin notes that the language in which these theories is presented indicates the difficulty of actually implementing them. The theorists constantly resort to metaphor: the assembly as map, mirror, portrait. It is difficult to even express the theory in more practical terms.

Mirroring the community may be as undesirable for selecting decision-makers as it is infeasible. The merriment that followed Senator Hruska's proposal that the mediocre deserved representation on the U.S. Supreme Court suggests a common understanding of the limits of simplistic views of descriptive representation.[19]

In addition, if representatives are asked merely to reflect the populace, they have no standards regarding their actions as representatives. Descriptive representation prescribes only who representatives should be, not what they should do.[20]

Though exacting microcosm theories are not realistic, descriptive standards are relevant to the operation of modern legislatures. Legislators are commonly criticized for not mirroring their constituents' views or interests. In fact, John Adams' formulation might be recast as one guideline to selecting representatives--the public votes, essentially, for candidates who appear to "think, feel, reason and act" as they do. But this broad conception of descriptive representation is sharply different from the utopian endeavor of forming a microcosm of the population in an assembly hall (or an HSA).

One contemporary version of the microcosm theory is what Greenstone and Peterson term "socially descriptive representation." Rather than mirroring opinions or interests, this conception proposes representational mirroring of the social and demographic characteristics of a community's population. A prevarious link is added to Adams' already rickety syllogism: if people (a) share demographic characteristics, (b) they will "think, feel and reason" like one another, and, (c) consequently, act like one another. Shared demographic characteristics, in this view, ensure like policy sentiments. This is both bad logic and pernicious to the substantive representation of consumer interests.

The problems with mirror theories, enumerated above, are all relevant to this version. Demographically mirroring a populace in an assembly is as unlikely as mirroring its opinions. Obviously, not all social characteristics can or ought to be represented. The problem of discriminating among them is particularly vexing. Common sense rebels against representing left-handers or redheads. What of Lithuanians? Italians? Jews? the uneducated? Mirror views provide few guidelines for selecting which social characteristics merit representation. Their central conception--the microcosm of society--is flawed, impossible.

Even when the characteristics to be mirrored are specified, problems remain. All individual members of a social group will not, in fact, "think, feel and reason" alike. And they will not represent with equal efficacy. Yet, by itself, mirror representation does not distinguish among members of a population group--one low-income representative is, for example, interchangeable with any other. As long as the requisite number of a population group is seated, the society is represented--mirrored--in the appropriate aspect. Such actors are not so much representatives as instances of population groups.

Socially descriptive representation is pernicious, because it makes recourse to constituencies unnecessary. The need for accountability and the careful specification of selection mechanisms is obviated. Skin color or income, for example, mark representatives acceptable or unacceptable, regardless of who selects them or what the constituency thinks. Consequently, any member of the group is as qualified a representative as any other. It is a situation that almost begs for tokenism. Where the only requirement is that a fixed percentage of a board be drawn from a specific group, there is nothing to recommend a black elected by fellow blacks or selected by the NAACP, or a woman, elected by women or selected by NOW, over blacks and women "drafted" onto a board because they will not "rock the boat."

Precisely this logic operated in the *Aldamuy* v. *Pirro* case, cited earlier. The court found no criteria in

either the original law or the regulations by which to
appraise the representativeness of the HSA board except
for descriptive characteristics. Since both the representatives of the board and their challengers satisfied the
criterion of minority status, there was no way to choose
between them. It was not possible to select one as any
better, or more representative, than another.

It has been suggested that socially descriptive representation might be effective if representatives were tied
to their constituencies by some mechanism of oversight.
That stipulation, however, moves beyond mere socially
descriptive representation. Selected agents are then
representatives not because they share a group's features,
but because they are acceptable to that group. P.L. 93-641,
as it was interpreted in the *Aldamuy* and *Texas Acorn*
(district level) cases, includes no such view. It requires
only that the composition of the board be a statistical
microcosm of the area's racial, social, linguistic, and
income distribution.

Still, for all its inadequacies, there is a "kernel of
truth" in theories of socially descriptive representation.
Obviously, social characteristics are sometimes related to
interests and, as the following section argues, interests
are precisely what ought to be represented. Thus, religious
affiliations bespeak clear interests in Northern Ireland,
race affects interests in America, and poverty relates to
interests everywhere. And while evaluating the actual
representation of interests (e.g., asking whether a board
cares about minorities) may be subtle and complex, toting
up the social categories attached to interests (e.g., how
many minorities are on their board?) is almost correspond-
ingly easy. The point of this section has been to show
that that is not sufficient to expand the health policy
role of overlooked groups.

Substantive Representation

The key issue in substantive representation is not what
representatives look like, but who they look after, whose
interests they pursue. Put simply, substantive representation means *acting in the interests of constituencies*.
Doing so involves both properly apprehending those interests
and effectively pursuing them.

The classic problem of ascertaining interests is immediately apparent.[21] Are interests objective facts that

intelligent leaders can best discern? Or are they more
like subjective preferences that must be conveyed to representatives? The latter requires a delegatory view, where
representatives follow constituent wishes. A more objective view of interests supports a trustee role, representatives acting in the constituent's best interest regardless
of their desires. In practice, substantive representation
involves neither of these extremes. Representatives are
neither unabashed messengers nor unfettered guardians for
interests. They are not completely objective or merely
subjective.

The nature of interests are easily caricatured in health
politics. Health policy is often technical and complex.
The guardian role is most often assumed not by the consumer representatives, but by health professionals, accountable to professional norms rather than consumers' desires.
The claim that they know the consumer's best interest is
accurate, but only within the confines of the physician's
office. For the issues that HSAs confront--such as the
distribution of limited resources among competing, needy
claimants--trusteeship on the basis of medical knowledge
is inappropriate.

As a matter of practical politics, representatives must
regularly consider demands to represent matters other than
constituency interests that this formulation stresses.
And precisely what is represented varies with the formal
setting and relevant function--members of a blue ribbon
commission, for example, might represent opinions more than
interests.

The effectiveness of representatives is crucial to substantive representation. An eloquent speaker or a skillful political operator can be said to provide better substantive representation than another with an equal understanding of constituent interests but without the same
skills. And representatives in influential positions--
chairs of congressional committees, officers of HSA
boards--may well be more effective than less well-placed
representatives. The reverse, representatives in positions
of little influence, can provide only minimal substantive
representation. A largely submerged issue for HSAs per-
tains to precisely this point. If HSAs are powerless and
inconsequential bodies, the furor over representation is
misplaced--consumer interests are substantively represented
within the HSAs but not in matters of important health
policy.

In sum, substantive representation means effectively acting in a constituency's interest. It is a concept that can guide all democratic representing, a measure by which any representative can be judged. The substantive view contrasts sharply with descriptive theories. To take one example, minorities are descriptively represented when minority representatives sit on an HSA board: they are substantively represented if board members (regardless of race) effectively pursue their interest. Crucially, final judgment about whether their interest has, in fact, been pursued must lie with the constituency. Either directly or indirectly, that minority constituency must control some mechanism (usually votes) by which to judge the policy that representatives have made in their name.

Some theorists have suggested that specific acts can be in a constituency's interest regardless of whether they concur; nevertheless--and regardless of the merits of this long disputed claim--designing representational systems is different from evaluating specific acts of representation. Ultimately, it is the constituency that ought to decide the disputed questions. This returns us to the topic of accountability: properly instituted substantive representation must rest on properly instituted mechanisms of accountability. The means by which this can be accomplished is the subject of the formal aspect of representation.

Formal Representation

Formal representation is the institutionalization of representation--the specific mechanisms by which representatives are selected and controlled. The mechanisms need have nothing to do with what representatives should be like (descriptive), or the way in which they should act (substantive). Yet they are crucial in defining the process of representation. They are the structure through which representation is established and carried on; they define constituencies and link representatives to them. Institutionalizing accountability rests in large measure on formal requirements. Likewise, moving from a descriptive to a substantive notion of representation is accomplished via formal mechanisms of representation.

One commonsense definition of representation is purely formal. Birch, for example, suggests that "the essential character of political representatives is the manner of

their selection, not their behavior or characteristics or
symbolic value."[22] To him, elections equal representation. Few theorists would agree to so starkly formal a
view. More commonly, elections must not merely be held
but must offer significant "choice"--they must be "free".[23]

Although empirical referents are often noted (elections
in the UK, not in the USSR), theorists have had difficulty
in specifying precisely what constitutes "free" elections.

The most important issue of formal representation relevant to P.L. 93-641 has been whether representatives should
be selected in general elections, by organized groups, by
officials, or by self-selection.

The health planning act has left most formal representational questions to be answered on the local level. This
is not necessarily unfortunate, as long as the applications
for designation are carefully reviewed regarding the issues
of formal representation. These issues can be stated in
broad terms by asking what constituency a representative
is tied to, and by what institutional arrangements.

Representation and the National Health Planning Act

The only passage in P.L. 93-641 relevant to representation
(in either the law or the regulations) mandated that consumers be "broadly representative of the social, economic,
linguistic, and racial characteristics of the population,"
a phrase that, conceptually, entitled every social group
that might want to sue for a place on a local HSA board.
And it set many HSAs to the misguided task of mirroring
whatever populations somehow seemed relevant or could
muster the influence. Formal representation--how representatives were to be selected--was not even mentioned.
In many places, representation was reduced, predictably,
to filling out complex grids of demographic characteristics. Accountability to local constituencies, overlooked
in the law and regulations, was seldom a concern. In short,
P.L. 93-641 left the HSAs mired in socially descriptive
representation.

The drafters of the original health planning act confused representativeness with substantive representation.
Mistakenly believing that socially descriptive representation would lead to effective representation of interests.
They presumed that a local agency with a jurylike board
would adequately represent the interests of consumers
and legitimate their regulatory interventions in the medical care market. Although jurylike bodies serve a

representative and legitimating function in some governmental contexts--notably determinations of guilt in criminal
trials--their capacity for substantive representation of
interests in circumstances requiring problem-solving
and complex conflict resolution is limited.

The amendments to the planning act (P.L. 96-79) introduce considerable improvement, largely through two changes.
The representational mandate is rewritten: from "broadly
representative of the social, economic, linguistic and
racial...populations of the area" to "broadly representative of the health service area and...including individuals
representing the social, economic, linguistic, handicapped
and racial populations of the area."[24] A grammatical
change reflects the conceptual difference: in the original
law, representation was an adjective describing individuals;
in P.L. 96-79, it is a verb, describing their behavior.
The law now calls for representatives of (very roughly)
specified constituencies rather than instances, or representations, of population groups.

Crucially, the change in language accompanies a mandate
that one-half the board members be chosen by some entity
other than the HSA. This requirement explicitly forces
HSAs to confront the issues of formal representation.
Rather than simply selecting board members to fit demographic requirements (as two-thirds of the HSAs had been
doing),[25] they must devise a process which grants some
entity within the community some accountability over some
of the board members. This statute change is important,
but partial for the local agencies are left to devise
their own process--and it only applies to half of the
board. It is certainly possible that mainly the provider
representatives will be selected by external entities, ensuring accountability and substantive representation for
provider constituencies while retaining descriptive representation for most consumers.

On balance the statute is improved. Mere microcosm
representation is no longer called for, formal representation and accountability are recognized and partially
mandated. But the amendments stopped short of issuing
clear, direct changes; change is left, rather, to local
HSAs. They are given tremendous latitude in how to structure formal representation and accountability and whom to
extend it to.

WHO IS TO BE REPRESENTED: A PRESCRIPTION

Only one representational category is precisely delineated
in the planning act--the public in nonmetropolitan areas
must be represented on the board in proportion to their
population.

Otherwise, the National Health Planning Act cut representation loose from geography; representatives stand for
social groups rather than precincts. However, the liberal-
ism that provides the theoretical foundation of the act
incorporates a vision of shifting cross-cutting interests
that makes it impossible to name functional categories
that enfranchise everyone equally. No matter what the
representational categories, some groups will gain, others
lose.

Difficult choices were avoided, in the original version
of the law, by entitling all population groups to repre-
sentation--a sweeping grant implicit in the microcosm
view. Representational categories were only vaguely specified. The result was considerable litigation.

The change in the language of the consumer representation
provision will reduce claims that a population group has
too few (or too many) representatives than is warranted by
their proportion of the population. But while the legal
terminology no longer evokes a microcosm, the precise
constituent categories--exactly *who* is represented--remains
vague.

If constituencies remain vague, confusion about who
represents whom and why is likely to persist. What aspect
of the health service area should consumers be "broadly
representative" of? Unscrambling present difficulties
requires an assessment of what consumer representation is
intended to accomplish. Presumably, the goal is to facilitate the articulation and satisfaction of the health
care needs in American communities. The reason for by-
passing normal politics, for cutting representation loose
from geography, is to enhance the interests that local
political processes often overlook. The reason for including such groups as minorities, low-income persons, and
women on the board should not be to mirror the community's
population on the boards (as the law originally attempted).
Rather, certain groups--minorities, low-income people, and
women--should be included, insofar as they have different
and important health interests that the political system
ought to consider.

The interests to be represented ought to be specified
on the federal level, in the regulations to the act.
Allowing local politics to define constituencies is fraught
with trouble. Note the cycle: Congress, claiming that
many interests were shut out of local politics, established
entirely new governmental structures for health planning
and mandated that they be "broadly representative."
That requirement is itself so broad that it is unclear
what interests qualify; the decision is left to the local
political process that Congress sought to bypass in the
first place. Still, the new language is an improvement,
for it breaks the cycle of litigation. Formerly, interests
that had been shunned could sue, arguing that the local
process that excluded them did not conform to the federal
mandate. Finally, there is a trade-off between competing
values; empowering unarticulated interests with federal
regulation versus local community control. This is exactly
the issue between Jefferson and Hamilton referred to above.

The next obvious question, then, is what specific consumer health interests should be represented on the HSA
board? The answer is not easy because interests vary by
issue. Regarding access to health care, for example, there
are different problems for rural and urban populations, or
for the chronically as opposed to the intermittently ill.

The infirm could claim representation for each of their
diseases whenever the issue of new facilities arises.
So could every ethnic group regarding specific genetic
diseases that disproportionately or exclusively afflict
them. The list of health interests is theoretically very
long. Note, however, that there are groups that, while
part of the population (and therefore potentially included
on a board constituted on the microcosm principle), do
not have distinctive health care interests. For example,
it is not clear that those with little formal education
have the distinguishable health needs that characterize
the low-income or aged populations. Congress (or its
delegate, HEW, must make these difficult choices and specify the various health interests that merit representation
on HSA boards.

As an illustration of interest selection, consider the
following representational categories. Although there is
no inherent symmetry or formal relationship among the
categories, there is a plausible, *a priori* justification
for representation of the following interests on HSAs:

(a) Payors. The most pressing issue in health politics
is rising costs. The interest with the clearest stake in
controlling them are the aggregated health care payors--
unions, large employers, insurance companies. In traditional markets, consumers are payors, but the dominance
of indirect or third-party health payors has necessitated
the distinction between payor and patient. Excluding the
former is likely to result in biased boards, for payors
have a clearly articulated financial interest that conflicts
directly with that of most health care providers.

(b) The poor. Reducing health services to control expenditures threatens groups that now receive insufficient
care, most obviously the poor. Their interests--more and
better care--are in conflict with those of the payors.
Providing board positions for advocates of the poor may
activate group interests that are difficult to organize
and thus, often overlooked.

(c) Racial minorities. Many racial minorities have the
same difficulty receiving adequate medical care as the
poor, because of poverty or discrimination, or as a result
of both.

(d) The elderly. The old rely on health services more
than any other age group. Despite a clear interest in
medical care, their concerns about access, quality, and
cost are easily overlooked in local politics.

(e) Women. Women require a different mix of health care
services from men. They too have clear health care interests that are not represented due to their near-exclu-
sion from local political processes.

(f) Catchment areas. Most health planning issues are,
at bottom, issues of geography--where to introduce a new
service or shut down an old hospital. Health interests
in these instances are unambiguous. With the exception
of the criteria for metropolitan and rural representation,
the planning act does attempt to replace areal with functional representation. But the two are not incompatible.
Indeed, the empirical evidence suggests that geographic
categories are emerging on many boards as counties, towns,
and neighborhoods win representatives. To carry the process
further, each HSA area could be broken into large catchment areas corresponding to the distribution of hospitals
and health services. Representatives could be drawn
from the various areas in approximate proportion to the
population.

(g) Special interests. There should also be a miscel-
laneous category for interests that form a significant

segment of an HSA's population--migrant workers, black lung victims, persons exposed to occupational hazards. These interests would be specified by the secretary of DHHS, either on the recommendation of the state or by appeal of the special interest. However, it is crucial that this be recognized as a residual category, filled by discretion of the secretary, not as a sweeping grant of representation to interests that count themselves a significant segment of some population.

Numerous objections can be raised to this specification of health interests that deserve representation on HSA boards.[26] People representing these interests may not value health in the same way as those having the same objective characteristics--whether they be related to sex, income, or minority status. They may also be members of a wide variety of groups, each with partially conflicting interests. This leads to two distinct problems: first, the temptation to multiply the number of interest groups represented until the board becomes unmanageable, and second, the tendency for representatives to neglect to speak for those interests that might be shared.

Admittedly, the notion of consumer interests in health is crude. And while we can state that some provider interests work against the interests of all consumers, we cannot unambiguously specify consumer interests as such due to their diversity.

But this diversity of consumer interests is itself the strongest argument for interest-based representation as a necessary, if not sufficient, condition for substantive representation of consumers. Without the quasi-corporatist amalgamations that interest representation can engender, consumer interests will simply not be pursued.

Naming specific representational categories will resolve some political and legal confusion. However, it suggests a deeper dilemma. As the proposed categories illustrate, the public is not neatly divisible into broad, roughly equivalent functional categories. How then can an HSA claim legitimacy to act as a public body when it does not equally enfranchise the entire population?

The answer is clear when there is a macrotheory of objective interests spanning the entire citizenry, such as class analyses include. However, liberal theory offers no comparable vision of fixed systematic interests. That does not mean, however, that we have no rationale for selecting legitimate interests.

Following Anderson, I suggest two criteria for assessing the legitimacy of such quasi-corporatist boards in a liberal setting.[27] First, the criteria for representation must be embedded in the board's function. Who is seated depends on what the body is expected to accomplish. Policy goals guide the selection of representational categories and constituencies. Interests are granted representation because it is reasonable to include them, given the nature and goals of the program. Within this rubric, particular attention might be paid to interests that past politics have subordinated despite the importance of health programs to them.

More important, however, legitimacy does not flow from elaborate representational schemes. HSAs are administrative agencies, established by Congress. Their legitimacy to act as public bodies lies in that legislative mandate. Functional representation schemes may stave off provider dominance, promote sensitivity to previously overlooked interests, or engender some accountability to local groups; but such achievements make HSAs no more or less legitimate than other congressional initiatives. Ultimately, geographic majoritarianism is supplemented, not supplanted.

Of course, designation of interests deserving representation is only one part of the resolution of representational difficulties in HSAs. Another part relates to the mechanisms that will guarantee substantive and accountable representation. The treatment of such policies follows the discussion of political imbalance and health issues.

IMBALANCED POLITICAL ARENAS

The puzzles of representation are exacerbated in circumstances that stimulate representation without explicitly structuring it--where there are no elections, no clearly defined channels of influence, or only vague conceptions of constituency. The politics of regulatory agencies or regional authorities provide examples of these circumstances. Though representatives of groups commonly press their interests within such contexts, there are no systematic canvasses of relevant interests such as are provided by geographically based elections. It is unclear who legitimately merits representation or how representation should be organized and operated.[28]

Interest group theorists address the problems of representation in precisely such political settings. In their view, unrepresented interests that are harmed coalesce and seek redress through the political system. Despite the absence of electoral mechanisms of representation, the theorists' conception of representation is universalistic; every interest that is strongly felt can organize a group to speak for it. And, at their most sanguine, group theorists suggest that "all legitimate groups can make themselves heard at some crucial stage in the decision-making process."[29] Politics itself, in this view, is characterized by legions of groups, bargaining at every level of government about policies that affect them. Government is viewed as the bargaining broker, policy choices as the consequences of mutual adjustment among the bargaining groups.

The group model is now partially in eclipse among political scientists.[30] One criticism is relevant here: groups that organize themselves for political action form a highly biased sample of affected interests.[31] Furthermore, that bias is predictable and recurs on almost every level of the political process. It is referred to as a tendency toward imbalanced political arenas, the unequal representation of equally legitimate but differentially affected interests.

Imbalance is present in part because organizing for political action is difficult and costly. Even if considerable benefits are at stake, potential beneficiaries may choose not to pursue them. If collective goods are involved (that is, if they are shared among members of a group regardless of the costs any other member paid to attain them, e.g., clean air), potential beneficiaries often let other members of the collectivity pay the costs and simply enjoy the benefits—the classic "free rider" problem.

Free riders aside, the probability of political action can be expected to vary with the material incentives. If either the benefits or costs of political action are concentrated, political action is more likely. A tax or a tariff on tea, for example, clearly and significantly affects the tea industry. To tea consumers, the tax is of marginal importance, a few dollars a year perhaps. Obviously, the former, with their livelihood at stake, are more likely to organize for political action, though even they are most likely to act if expected benefits outweigh costs. "The clearer the material incentives of the organization's members, the more prompt, focused and vigorous the action."[32]

The most common stimulant to group organization is threat to occupational status, as observers of American politics from de Toqueville to David Truman have argued. If the group model overstated the facility and extent of group organization, some of its proponents isolated the most significant factor: narrow, concentrated producer interests are more likely to pay the costs of political action than broad, diffuse consumer interests.

Not only do concentrated interests have a larger incentive to engage in political action, they act with two significant advantages. First, they typically have ongoing organizations with staff and other resources available. This dramatically lowers the marginal cost of political action. Secondly, most organizations have an expertise that rivals other political interests, even government agencies. Their superior grasp, and sometimes monopoly, of relevant information translates into political influence. The more technical an area, the more powerful the advantage, but it is almost always present to some extent.

In sum, two phenomena work to imbalance political arenas: unequal interests and disproportionate resources. The two are interrelated--groups with more at stake will invest more to secure an outcome. However, the distinction warrants emphasis for it has important policy implications. Attempts to stimulate countervailing powers by making resources available to subordinate groups will fail if they do not account for differing incentives in their employment. For example, even a resource such as equal access to policymakers (now the goal of considerable political effort) is meaningless if the incentives to utilize it over time are grossly unequal. The reverse case--equal interests, unequal resources--is too obvious to require comment. But that clarity should not obscure the fact that the dilemma of imbalance is deeper than the obvious inequality of group resources suggests.

Naturally, diffuse consumer interests are not always somnolent. There are purposive as well as material incentives to political action. A revolt against a sales tax might necessitate cuts in programs that benefit specific groups--diffuse payors defeating concentrated beneficiaries. Tea drinkers may be swept into political action, even to the point of dumping tea into Boston Harbor. Both are examples of diffuse interest uniting for political

action. Such coalitions tend to have a grass roots style
of organization. Since sustained, long-term political
action requires careful organization, they tend to be
temporary. With the end of political deliberation, the
group disbands or sets out in search of new issues. Concentrated interests, however, carry on, motivated by the
same material incentives that first prompted political
action.

The advantages of organized groups increase after a
policy's inception. Such groups can be expected to pursue the policy through its implementation and administration. Administrative politics are far less visible than
legislative. They are not bounded by discrete decisions
and they are cluttered with technical detail rather than
the emotive symbols likely to arouse diffuse constituencies. The policy focus of program administration is dis-
persed temporally, conceptually, even geographically.
Concentrated groups are much more likely to sustain a
commitment to participate.

Administrative processes may even grow biased to the
point that other affected parties are shut out from deliberations that concern them. Important decisions are made
in agencies and bureaus that define, qualify, or even sub-
vert original legislative intent. For example, Congress
included a consumer participation provision in the Hill-
Burton Act, but the implementing agency never wrote the
regulations for it. When consumers overcame the imbalance
of interests and sued for participation, they were denied
standing. Since the regulations had never been written,
consumer representatives had no entry into the policymaking process.[33]

The major question for HSAs is how to overcome these
tendencies and balance the politics of health or even promote consumer control. Both the law's emphasis on participation, and the political economy of health all point to
a continuation of imbalanced health planning arenas.
HSAs were created to exert control over health providers;
political theory would predict that the major issue concerning their governing boards is how to avoid provider
domination.

REPRESENTING CONSUMER INTERESTS: OVERCOMING THE POLITICAL
OBSTACLES

The task is overcoming political imbalance rather than
just getting consumers on health planning boards. This

section suggests how more effective representation of and accountability to local health interests might be established.

The HSA staffs could help consumers achieve political parity. Staffs have considerable expertise in issues of medical care and health. Occupying full-time positions in health planning, they have a concentrated interest in the industry. If they ally with providers, or fail to take consumers seriously, they will easily undermine consumer representatives who cannot match the combined expertise of providers and staff. The support of the staff is essential to an active consumer role on HSA boards. The problem is systematically harnessing the staffs' market balancing potential to consumer interests.

The 1979 amendments take an important step in the direction. They require that "at least one member of the staff shall be designated to...provide the members of the governing body...(particularly the consumer members) with such information and technical assistance as they may require to effectively perform their functions."[34] The importance of such professional (i.e., expert, full-time) support to the consumer effect cannot be overstated. And, even stronger language would have been preferable. The Senate version, for instance, assigned staff support to consumer members alone. And, optimally, that staffer would be directly under consumer control--selected by and accountable to them. Nevertheless, this is an important improvement for consumer representation.

Another potential for balancing the health planning market lies in organizations that already exist within the consumer population.[35] They should select consumer board members. The very existence of these groups attests to a commitment to enhance the life circumstances of some part of the population. Furthermore, they have already paid the costs of organizing. We can expect them to devote attention to issues in a relatively sustained manner; and they can often overcome low expertise by redeploying their staff. Representatives from these groups will have clearly defined, and often attentive, constituencies, experience in organizational politics and resources at their disposal. These attributes will help them both in identifying group interests and in pursuing them, regardless of their other descriptive characteristics. Even minorities suing for representation in Texas, for example, were willing to accept whites representing blacks if the NAACP selected them. It is telling that much of the litigation

challenging HSA boards comes from organizations formed
to further the rights or general circumstances of disadvantaged groups within the consumer population.

The historical evidence supports this contention. The
poverty boards of the 1960s (particularly the War on
Poverty's Community Projects), for example, tended to be
most capable when their members were selected by organizations.

Ideally, then, the imbalanced political features of
health planning will be tempered by two mechanisms, one
internal to the Health Systems Agency (staff assigned to
the consumer representatives), the other external (selection of representatives by groups). The former will facilitate organization and expertise among the consumer representatives, the latter improve substantive representation
and heighten accountability.

Note that both these recommendations are (at least) facilitated by P.L. 96-79. Staff is explicitly assigned to
the board (and particularly the consumers). And with self-
selection limited, a large majority of the HSAs will need
to devise new selection procedures for at least part of
their governing board. DHHS would do well to urge the
use of organized groups in local selection processes.

Various other modes of selection (or formal representation) have been suggested. I evaluate two others:
general elections and selection by officials.

General Elections. Various reform groups have called for
election of consumer representatives in a model roughly
based on the selection of school boards. The surface
plausibility of the proposal should not be permitted to
obscure its difficulties. One problem with direct election of representatives to HSA boards stems from the failure of most Americans to consider themselves part of an
ongoing health care community. They typically seek care
sporadically, and do not conceive of health care in terms
of local systems. Both factors distinguish health planning from education or housing issues where specific elections may be more effective.

Evidence from other programs supports the view that
elections are problematic: less than 3 percent of the
eligible population voted for local poverty boards in
Philadelphia; less than 1 percent voted in Los Angeles.
Those who did vote were moved to do so by personal, not
policy, considerations. Overwhelmingly, they voted for
neighbors and personal acquaintances. The policy formulated

by these representatives was, predictably, particularistic. It helped their friends, not the community or the interests they ostensibly represented. Representatives generated little community interest or support. They tended to be ineffective advocates.

The evidence from HSAs that have held elections is strikingly similar--low turnout at the polls and high turnover among representatives. Representatives are uncertain of their task and their constituency. Furthermore, direct elections have facilitated the takeover of entire boards by single organizations. In northeastern Illinois, for example, abortion foes captured the HSA, linking every health concern to their own preoccupation; in Illinois, Arkansas, and Massachusetts, provider institutions chartered buses and flooded the polling places with hospital workers who voted for docile consumer representatives.[36]

Elections are appealing to reformers because they permit the public to choose health planning representatives directly; theoretically, the representatives can be held accountable with relative ease. In practice, the low incentives (predicted by the theory of imbalanced markets) and marginal visibility will undermine direct elections as a mechanism of accountability to consumer constituencies.

Selection by Local Officials. This mechanism leaves accountability to the public very tenuous. The constituency is left with no direct control over its representatives, but must hold the selector of the representatives to account. In the worst cases, the selector is not directly accountable to the public either. Boards selected by local officials are accountable to, and presumably controlled by, local government; they will be as accountable as any other local agency. Yet they operate within a program that promises direct consumer participation. When a health planning issue becomes highly visible, we expect this mismatch of rhetoric and reality to cause public frustration and alienation.

Since officials can choose whichever member of a group they desire, many will choose ones that "make no trouble." Thus, descriptive representation (what representatives "think, feel and reason") will probably be low even when socially descriptive representation is high.

Substantive representation will generally be low. The HSA, over time, will become indistinguishable from other agencies in the local health-care bureaucracy.

Still, this selection mode may have the advantage of erecting a formal link between the HSA and local government. The questions of legitimacy--likely to plague these peculiarly designed agencies--might thus be minimized. Theoretically, then, local government selection has some advantages; but it is less likely to produce substantive representation than the model recommended above--selection by organized groups.

LITIGATION

P.L. 93-641 triggered a spate of litigation, much of it turning on issues of consumer representation. The following cases illustrate some of the arguments I have made about representation and accountability--all were litigated prior to the health planning amendments.

Aldamuy et al. v. *Pirro et al.*, C.A. No. 76 CV-206 (N.D.N.Y., April 7, 1977). The plaintiff sued, arguing that they were more representative of Onedaga County's minority population than the minority representatives that had been seated on the HSA board. The court ruled against them; it found that if the requisite number of minority individuals were on the board, the law's mandate was fulfilled.

The court simply applied a mirror view of representation. It found no criterion in either the law or the regulations by which to judge representatives except for descriptive characteristics (in this case, "minority" status). Since both the representatives originally selected for the HSA board and their challengers satisfied that criterion, there was no way to choose between them; it was not possible to select one minority group member as any better, or more "representative," than any other. Since P.L. 93-641 and its regulations said nothing about the selection of representatives or their accountability to constituencies, challengers had no recourse if the minimal criterion of socially descriptive representation was satisfied. Under the 1979 amendments, the court would have had formal selection criteria by which to measure the contending groups. Though these are instituted locally, P.L. 96-79 requires that they be "open and participatory."

Texas ACORN et al. v. *Texas Area V Health Systems Agency et al.*, C.A. No. S-76-102-CA (E.D. Texas, Sherman Div., March 1, 1977). The plaintiffs argued that only 3 of the 41 consumer representatives had incomes below the mean

for the area ($10,000). They argued that if people with
income above the median were to represent low-income consumers, then the burden of proof was on the defendant HSA
to show how they do so.

The district court ruled that the HSA was improperly
constituted, that between 16 and 25 of the 41 representatives on the board of Texas Area V HSA must have incomes
below the area's mean--thus, a strictly mathematical de-
lineation was made with a little give in it to make it
"broadly" rather than precisely representative.

In this case the defendants are caught in socially descriptive representation. In bringing suit, the ACORN
organization used the mirror conception to their advantage. However, they recognized that it alone would not
suffice to produce adequate representation of consumer
interests over time. They acknowledged that clearly defined selection mechanisms may be more important than the
socially descriptive representational requirements that
made their litigation possible. They were willing to waive
socially descriptive criteria in favor of accountability
in the selection process. The trade-off was illustrated
in ACORN's brief with the suggestion that a white, selected
by the NAACP, would be acceptable from the perspective of
black interests.

Texas ACORN et al. v. *Texas Area V HSA et al.*, 559
F2nd 1019(U.S. Court of Appeals, 5th Circ., Sept. 23,
1977). On appeal, a broader view of this case was taken.
The district court's undifferentiated mirror view was
rejected and a full evidentiary hearing in which HEW could
demonstrate precisely how board members were representative
of the low-income population was mandated. The view that
to represent low-income or demographic populations one must
be a member of those groups was explicitly rejected.

This ruling appeared to show greater sensitivity to the
issues of representation. There appeared to be cognizance
of questions about the representatives' relationships to
their constituencies and the necessity of various skills
relevant to achieving substantive representation; in sum,
an awareness that a mindless adherence to the mirroring
view can undermine the effective representation of a constituency's interests.

The crucial issue in the hearing, of course, would be
what counts as evidence that high-income consumers are
properly representing low-income populations. The most
direct evidence would be acceptability to those populations, i.e., some manner of formal representation.

Amos et al. v. *Central California Health Systems
Agency et al.*, C.A. No. 76-174 ci (E.D. Calif., filed
Sept. 10, 1976). The plaintiffs charged that whites were
underrepresented on the board because Fresno and Kern
counties were underrepresented. HEW sent the defendant
agency a letter noting that the governing board did not
conform to the requirements of P.L. 93-641 because the
representation of metropolitan and nonmetropolitan populations was not fixed in exact proportion to the population. The race issue was not dealt with directly but
subsumed within the criticism of the board's geographic
representation. This case did not reach trial.

The *Amos* case illustrates two difficulties discussed
above. First, the charge that minorities "captured" this
HSA board recalls the distinction between (a) giving contending groups a place on the board and letting them dispute policy questions and (b) letting groups contend for
the places on, or control over, the board. The latter
defeats the purpose of representative boards that allow
local consumer interests to "hash out" local health issues
with each other as well as with providers. As originally
structured, the law invited attempts at this undesirable
"capture" by some consumer groups because it left the
crucial question of who is being represented (i.e., which
consumer interests) to the local political game.

Precisely who is being represented was not made clear
by a law and regulations that merely mandated broad representation of the "social, economic, linguistic, and racial
populations...of the health service area."

It was a meaningless guide to the selection of constituencies; and even the new amendments remain vague on
this subject. The interests that merit representation
must be specified precisely on the national level. This
case illustrates one reason why: geography is the one
representational category precisely specified by the law;
as a consequence, the *Amos* case was reduced from a difficult litigation to an administrative memorandum.

CONCLUSION

The National Health Planning Act's original vision of
representation was impossibly flawed, but not irretrievably
so. The 1979 amendments introduced considerable improvement. I have tried to evaluate the strengths and short-
comings of both the law and its amendments. Though the

changes are often partial and hesitant, they unquestionably strengthen the effort to represent local constituencies. Further improvements--for both local and national levels-- have been sketched out above. However, representing consumers, overcoming imbalance, even discerning the public interest on HSAs will not alter the American health system in any profound fashion. The HSA mandate--limiting costs, expanding access, and improving the quality of health--reaches far beyond the agency's capabilities. Measured by these standards, the act's program is trivial-- more symbols and rhetoric than significant improvement.

Rather, the law's significance lies in its stimulation of a broad range of consumer interests. Viewed as an effort to organize communities into caring for their own health systems, it is the largest program of its kind, and one that could influence health politics long after its particular institutional manifestation--HSA planning boards--have been forgotten.

NOTES

1. P.L. 93-641 §1512(b)(3)(c)(iii)(2).
2. *Aldamuy et al.* v. *Pirro et al.*, C.A. No. 76 Cv206 (N.D., N.Y., April 7, 1977).
3. *Texas Association of Community Organizations for Reform Now (ACORN) et al.*, UCA No. S-76-102-CA (E.D. Texas, Sherman Div., March 1, 1977).
4. *Rakestraw et al.*, v. *Califano et al.*, C.A. No. (77-635A N.D. Ga., Atlanta Div., filed April 22, 1977). *The Louisiana Association of Community Organizations for Reform Now (ACORN) et al.* v. *New Orleans Area/Bayou Rivers Health Systems Agency et al.*, C.A. No. 17-361 (E.D. La., filed March 15, 1977).
5. 41 *Federal Register* 12812 (March 26, 1976), §122.114.
6. *Ibid.*, §§122.104(b)(1)(viii) and 122.109(e)(3).
7. *Ibid.*, §§122.104(a)(8) and 122.104(b)(7).
8. *Ibid.*, §122.107(c)(2).
9. *Ibid.*, §122.107(c)(3).
10. This argument is elaborated and placed in the British context in Rudolf Klein in "Control, Participation and the British National Health Service, *Health and Society*, 57(1), 1979.
11. P.L. 93-641 §1515(c)(1).
12. H. F. Pitkin, *The Concept of Representation* (Berkeley: University of California Press, 1967), p. 3.

13. This is not so for certain groups, e.g., the parents of children with special diseases--as my colleague Owen Fiss points out.

14. T. R. Marmor, "Consumer Representation: Beneath the Consensus, Many Difficulties," *Trustee* 30(April 1977): 37-40.

15. Meetings may be closed if they deal with employees (and "would sonstitute a clearly unwarranted invasion of . . . privacy") or with "the agency's participation in a judicial proceeding." P.L. 96-70. §1512(B)(6)(A).

16. Pitkin, *The Concept of Representation*, p. 8.

17. This formulation originates with A. Phillips Griffiths, "How Can One Person Represent Another?" *Aristotelian Society*, Supplementary Volume 34, 1960. It was refined and popularized by Pitkin, *Concept of Representation, passim*.

18. John Adams, cited in Pitkin, *The Concept of Represenation*, p. 60.

19. For notable formulations of this common idea, see Edmund Burke, "The English Constitutional System," in Pitkin (ed.), *Representation* (New York: Atherton Press, 1969), or James Madison, *Federalist Paper,* Number 10 (New York: Modern Library, 1937).

20. Judged by the model of a jury, such standards are necessary; representativeness is the condition for legitimacy.

21. See Brian Barry, *Political Argument* (London: Rutledge and Kegan Paul, 1965), and Isaac Balbus, "The Concept of Interest in Pluralist and Marxian Analysis" in Ira Katznelson *et al.* (ed.), *The Politics and Society Reader* (New York: John Wiley & Sons, 1966).

22. Birch, A., *Representation* (New York: Praeger, 1971).

23. Friedrich, C. J., *Constitutional Government and Democracy* (New York: Blaisdell and Swabey, M.C., 1969), 266ff. "The Representative Sample" in Pitkin, H. F. (ed.), *Representation* (New York: Atherton Press).

24. P.L. 96-79 §1512(b)(3)(c)(i)(II).

25. Reported by Mark Kleiman, "What's in It for Us?" a consumer analysis of the 1979 Health Planning Amendments, *Health Law Project Library Bulletin* IV (Oct. 1979):333.

26. I have profiled particularly from Albert Weale's incisive comments on the topic of interests.

27. Charles Anderson, "Political Design and the Representation of Interests," *Comparative Political Studies* 10 (April 1977).

28. The problem is less nettlesome in legislatures. On a practical level, lobbying legislatures appears only

marginally effective: analysts have generally found that politicians are most likely to follow their own opinions or apparent constituency desires. More important, there is at least a formal representation of every voting citizen. Of course, this does not minimize the complexities of electoral representation. But elective systems do afford a systematic canvas of community sentiment, however vague a guide it may be to policy formulation.

29. Robert Dahl, *A Preface to Democratic Theory* (Chicago: The University of Chicago Press, 1964), p. 137.

30. See Andrew McFarland, "Recent Social Movements and Theories of Power in America," paper delivered at the American Political Science Convention, Washington, D.C., 1979.

31. Revall Schattschneider's epigram: "The flaw in the pluralist heaven is that the heavenly chorus sings with a strong upper class accent. Probably about 90 percent of the people cannot get into the pressure system." E. E. Schattschneider, *The Semisovereign People* (Hinsdale: The Dryden Press, 1960), p. 34.

32. James Q. Wilson, *Political Organizations* (New York: Basic Books, 1973), p. 318; T. R. Marmor and D. Wittman, "Politics of Medical Inflation," *Journal of Health Politics, Policy and Law* (Spring 1976).

33. Rand Rosenblatt, "Health Care Reform and Administrative Law, A Structural Approach," *Yale Law Journal* 1978, Part 2.

34. 1512(b)(2)(A).

35. See P. C. Schmitter, "An Inventory of Analytical Pluralist Propositions" (unpublished monograph, University of Chicago, Autumn, 1975).

36. C.f. Mark Kleiman, "What's in It for Us? A Consumer Analysis of the 1979 Health Planning Amendments," *Health Law Project Library Bulletin* IV(Oct. 1979):329-336, and Barry Checkoway, "Citizens on Local Health Planning Boards: What Are the Obstacles?" *Journal of the Community Development Society* X:101-116.

THE REAL WORLD OF REPRESENTATION: CONSUMERS AND THE HSAs

James A. Morone

In the early days of P.L. 93-641, an oft-voiced notion was that planning agencies would be dominated by provider governing body members, despite the statutorily required consumer majority. The vision of such pessimists has not been totally realized. In this paper Morone characterizes agency staff and provider and consumer board members of six Health Systems Agencies. He examines factors that encourage or inhibit effective consumer participation. In the last section of the paper he turns to project review activities, describing frustrations felt by board members, concluding that, as cost containers, consumers face considerable obstacles.

PREFACE*

Consumer representatives on Health Systems Agencies were expected to fail. Consumers would be bewildered by the

*The arguments presented here are based on site visits (averaging 10 days each) to the HSAs in: Philadelphia, Idaho, Atlanta, Minneapolis/St. Paul, Detroit, west-central Illinois. The agencies were selected to include differences in the following characteristics: geography, type of organization, selection of representatives, and impressions of effectiveness by observers of agencies. Over 100 respondents were interviewed; the interviews averaged very roughly 90 minutes. The conceptual foundations for the study are presented in some detail in "Models of Representation: Consumers and the HSAs," published in this volume.

technical complexities of health planning and dominated
by provider representatives. Drawn by the fanfare at the
program's initiation, consumers would soon be overwhelmed
and give up. The AMA declared that "two physicians on a
30 man board (could) sway decisions";[1] a conference of
academics and state officials in Florida thought it would
take only one.[2]

Some early reports confirmed the pessimists. Wayne
Clarke's widely read *Placebo or Cure?* depicted an almost
complete lack of meaningful consumer involvement: meetings
in which no consumers attended, chronic failure to achieve
quorum, and complete dominance by organized providers
characterized his sample of southern HSAs.[3]

Four years later, Clarke's bleak description no longer
applies. In the six HSAs visited for this report--includ-
ing one that Clarke tallied up as a dismal failure--there
was at least a core of active, knowledgeable consumers.
In Detroit and Minneapolis/St. Paul, most respondents
(consumers, staff, and providers) felt that consumers dominated; in Philadelphia and Atlanta they "hold their own";*
in Idaho, providers dominate--but not easily, not always
and there is a widespread sense of learning and improvement among "a core" of the consumer members. Consumer
representatives are developing considerable skill and
knowledge. They commit long hours (representatives in
Minnesota averaged 10 to 15 hours a week) and are generally
comfortable with the arcane HSA processes. In short, consumer representatives know a CON application from a PUFF
review.

The case can be overstated. In most places it is true
of the consumer leaders rather than the entire contingent.
And by all accounts the knowledge has often been acquired
"slowly and painfully" over the 5 years of the program.
Nevertheless, the consumer representation I observed in
Atlanta, for example, was strikingly different from the
thoroughgoing provider dominance described by Clarke and
recalled by some of my respondents). Almost every veteran
board member emphasizes how much has been learned. Consumer representation on HSAs has made an auspicious start.
Community members have become actively and knowledgeably
involved in their health care system. By these criteria
P.L. 96-79 is a success.

And yet, on a larger, programmatic level consumer

---

*All unascribed quotations are taken from interviews.

representation on P.L. 96-79 is troubled. My interviews were marked not only by the intelligence of the respondents but, often, a sense of futility, a lack of salience.

Despite the successes, this is not a sanguine report. The National Health Planning Act faces considerable, perhaps insurmountable problems. The expectations of the program far exceed its capabilities. And in many places, consumer advocacy in health is being measured for its epilogue, even while the relative success of consumer boards becomes clear.

Within these board parameters--successes and failures, unrealistic ambitions, and potential changes--this essay reports the experiences of six HSAs and their board members. I have sought, particularly, the common themes that typify HSAs in sites as divergent as Philadelphia and Idaho, Atlanta and central Illinois.

First, I suggest a typology of board members, particularly the different categories of consumers. Second, I take up a series of topics in representing consumers; I try to lay out some of the pieces that comprise the puzzling question: What makes for effective consumer representatives (and, how do you know when you have them)? Third, I sketch what I take to be the major difficulty of the National Health Planning Act--the tasks that the boards have been set to.

REPRESENTATIVES: A TYPOLOGY OF HSA ACTORS

This section examines the HSA actors. Discussions about them are often cast in sweeping terms--providers are said to be greedy, consumers gulled. This paper takes a closer look, suggesting some categories and distinctions. After some notes on the HSA staffs, I suggest a typology of provider reactions to health planning, then lay out a more detailed catalogue of consumer types.

Staff

Both analysts and activists looking for a fight in health planning flocked around the consumer/provider schism. The staff was largely overlooked--a resource, perhaps, for uneducated consumers, a potential balancer to provider expertise and vigor. In fact, the staff fundamentally alters the politics of the HSAs.

The HSA staffers are generally planning professionals.
They have graduate degrees and are recruited through
national searches--they are cosmopolites rather than locals. Both their legitimacy in the HSA process and their
view of it is rooted in their profession. All professionals are accountable, not to constituent desires but to
occupational norms--they answer to peers on the basis of
technical skill. Furthermore, those skills are generally
integrated into a larger vision, a set of attitudes that
are shaped by their professional role. For planners, that
"skill ideology" is marked by a rationalistic, systemic,
universalistic turn. They see interrelated populations
rather than single individuals.

Although governing boards (or their committees) make
policy decisions, they rely heavily on staff for analysis
and implementation. Often, staff domination is a concern.
Reflecting this worry, some agencies request that their
staff avoid making recommendations and simply report
"findings of facts" when discussing certificate-of-need
projects. (An epistimologically untenable distinction,
perhaps, but one that illustrates the sensitivity of the
dominance issues.)

Staff-board relations vary widely. The staff is visibly
deferential in many HSAs, their roles unambiguously pre-
scribed--assisting the board (e.g., Idaho, west-central
Illinois). In other agencies, there is a comfortable division of labor, though less deference (Minneapolis-St.
Paul). And in still others the relationship is ill defined
and occasionally conflicting. Detroit had been the extreme case; they spent extraordinary time and energy
trying to untangle their board-staff relationship (though
in that anomolous case board domination of staff was at
issue). Of the six agencies studied, three had no such
problems; and all of them had fired at least one executive
director.

Often (in four of six sites) the staff members were
less comfortable with political issues than technical
ones. The latter is a perspective that minimizes conflict,
even when it contains unabashedly political implications.
Staff may be accused of "being wedded to its numbers,"
but arguments are bounded by clearly recognized roles.
When both sides regard the other as "political" (generally
a charge leveled at the top staff), clashes occur more
frequently, and are more intense.

In any case, staff generally combat provider dominance
of HSAs. They tend to cultivate the consumer board members

more than the providers. Consumers are most likely to
concur with their technical systemwide, regulatory
outlook and the recommendations (or the findings of fact)
that follow from it. However, this staff outlook is more
suited to some HSA functions than others. It generally
does not prepare staff to promote broad-based citizen
participation, though in some cases staff members with
community organizing skills are hired specifically for
them. Even where this is so, it is the participatory and
advocacy HSA functions that tend to be sacrificed for the
regulatory/rationalizing ones.[4] Some consumers are particularly critical of this choice. Charges of "provider
dominance" generally follow.

Provider domination of staff seemed a reasonable pre-
diction, but it did not characterize any of the agencies
I studied. An articulated government interest distinguishes the HSA case from classic cases of agency "capture." The steady lobbying of the industry is steadily
opposed by DHHS. The latter reinforces precisely the
rationalistic/regulatory values that professional planners
are likely to hold (and industry lobbyists likely to
fight).

Much enthusiasm has greeted the realization that staffs
comprise a reasonable antidote to provider dominance.
However, despite the relative good will they often show
consumers, their critics score an important point: ultimately professional planners embody the antithesis of
citizen representation. Models of community participation
are generally founded on an urge to counter traditional
reform values such as professionalism, universalism, and
rationalization--the very essence of the planning vision.

Providers

Physicians, too, operate within a professional ethic; much
of their legitimacy on HSAs flows from their expertise.
However, their outlook contrasts sharply with the staff's
universalism; it is intensely individualistic. As physicians, they are expected to apply every resource at their
disposal toward the individual before them. There is no
conception of opportunity costs, pareto optimality, or
the rationing of scarce resources; and hospital administrators perceive individual institutions, not health
systems. Thus, staff and provider paradigms are exactly
contrary: a system view versus an individualistic one.

Much of the heat of board politics is generated by the
clash of these antithetical visions.

Within this framework, there are various provider perspectives on health planning. Four "types" are typical of
HSA provider activists around the country:

1. Neanderthal. Government has no place in medicine.
Neanderthals often join boards explicitly to capsize them.
The American Medical Association placed itself solidly in
this category by urging Congress to overturn the National
Health Planning Act, while suggesting pointedly that its
members participate in the program.[5]

2. Self-Seekers. Providers (often administrators) who
use planning to their own (institution's) ends. The classic
maneuver is to get a certificate of need for your expansion, then oppose a competitor's. The strategy requires
a provider community that has abandoned solidarity; a
vital peak association generally indicates where that solidarity remains. (Thus, the Greater Detroit Hospital Council has subordinated advocacy to other functions, while the
Delaware Valley Hospital Council or the Idaho Hospital Association actively represent their members before government
bodies.)

After unsuccessfully opposing regulation, industries have
often embraced it to defend entrenched interests. And
certificate of need is well designed to bar potential
competitors. In this case, it can provide a strong show
of planning--projects turned down, dollars saved--while
undermining its essence, i.e., a systematic assessment and
pursuit of community health needs.[6]

3. Tory. A tory response is cautious reform to avert
revolutionary change. A spot of health planning might
solve--admitted--problems less painfully than a federal
program of health insurance or cost containment. Tories
seem to be integral to well-functioning governing boards.

4. Renegade. Dedicated to health planning or cost
containment or other innovation that might alter the
organization, financing, or practice of medicine. Renegades
have abandoned the highly individualistic perspective that
characterizes all the preceding categories; like planners,
they perceive health in system terms.

These categories refer largely to physicians and administrators. However, many other provider occupations are
active on HSAs. Many of these nonelite providers fit less
in provider categories than consumer ones. Thus, providers

serving the underprivileged often become their advocates;
nurses are likely to develop a perspective indistinguishable from the Volunteers described below; and in their
fight for health system legitimacy, physician extenders,
midwives, even chiropractors may ally closely with consumer factions. They are far more likely to be Tories or
Renegades than other providers.

Tellingly, consumer activists often seek to rearrange
provider HSA seats by increasing the numbers of "allied
health professionals" (e.g., midwives, nurse-extenders).
Still, the role of these actors is sometimes overstated;
the bedrock interest of the most visible HSA providers
remains lodged in the present structure, financing, and
organization of medical care.

Consumers, of course, draw legitimacy from representing
constituencies rather than professional skills. A great
many generalizations are made about "HSA consumers." In
reality, there are some very distinctive types. Ask HSA
activists (of any type) about consumers and they almost
inevitably respond--"Well, there are consumers and there
are *consumers.*" I found the following types of consumers:

1. Eminents and Warm Bodies. These are the representatives who fulfill the expectations of consumer representation's cynics and critics.

Faced with the task of filling consumer representative
seats, many HSAs sought local notables. Well-known lawyers,
city council members, university deans were "drafted" for
community service. At first blush it seemed a plausible
strategy, reflecting the fashion in building corporate
boards. However, HSA representatives face a tremendous
workload of technically complex issues (itself an issue,
discussed below); treating board membership as yet another
honorific service leads to inadequate preparation and uncertain participation. Many Eminents are simply too busy.
Others are not sufficiently interested. They rarely understand what board membership entails when they join.

Variation in the eminence theme are common. Agencies
sometimes decide they need a mix of skills; engineers,
architects, or--who knows--locksmiths are sought with the
same results. In another variant, individuals join the
boards for prestige (or eminence); "it gets them a paragraph in the local paper." This variant remains common,
even where HSAs seek to recruit hard workers rather than
eminent names.

In any case, Eminents fill out an agency roster but contribute little. Their numbers vary--considerably--from agency to agency. They are more likely to sit on governing boards than executive committees. And they are often the product of self-selecting boards (in the case of drafted Eminents) or very loose selection procedures such as elections (eminence seekers).

Naturally, board members originally in this category may develop an interest in HSA activity and make substantial contributions. However, those that do so have jumped categories [usually to Volunteers (2)]. Eminents are defined by their minimal contribution. Wayne Clarke's recital of consumer bewilderment in southern HSAs was largely about this category of consumer.

Warm Bodies share the same fundamental characteristics-- minimal contribution. The descriptive mandate and some legal interpretations of P.L. 93-641 sent agencies scrambling for "x minorities, $x + 1$ aged and a half a dozen senior citizens." Representation is reduced to a demographic sampler. Many agencies evince this mindlessly descriptive approach (reinforced by constant badgering from DHHS' regional office). When asked if the poor are well represented, the answer is often framed in terms of "Warm Bodies": "Our percentages of income (racial, age) groups are OK." Questions about ability or acceptability to constituency are not considered. Theorists had asked how individual HSAs would deal with the impossible mandate to "broadly represent social, economic, linguistic and racial populations . . . of the . . . area." The answer is clear: they tallied up the Warm Bodies that they thought that DHHS would think were relevant. A major question about the changes in language introduced by the planning amendments will be how it changes HSA approaches to representing specific interests like the poor. They may increasingly ignore them; or the limit on self-perpetuating boards may lead HSAs to turn accountability over to the relevant groups; or the hunt for Warm Bodies and a statistical reflection of the census tract may remain.

Note, finally, that the structures of many HSAs accommodate, even promote, a large number of do-nothings, whether Eminents, Warm Bodies, or some other sort: large governing boards, often, meet only four times a year to "rubber stamp executive committee decisions" (and never even see certificate-of-need projects).

2. Volunteers. Essentially advocates without a cause,
Volunteers join the HSAs seeking to do some communal good.
They take a universalistic perspective--some variant of
the public interest--eschewing narrow interest constituencies. Their major point of reference is not a health
system goal (like Advocates (3) or a constituency [Inter-
est Group Champions (4)], but the entire community, perceived through the HSA and its process. (They almost
always speak of the agency as "we.")

Since they join HSA with relatively weak health system
ideologies, Volunteers tend to assume the rationalistic,
systemic one that characterizes most HSA staffs. It is an
outlook that fits neatly with their universalistic perspective. They are generally the staff's strongest ally.
At the same time, Volunteers generally exhibit a noncon-
flicting style, they are the board members most likely to
get along with all the factions on the HSA. Community
notables who become active in the agency generally fit
into this Volunteer category.

Volunteers demonstrate many of the traits often as-
cribed to such "voluntary associations" as hospital boards
and mental health associations. After World War II, these
groups were " . . . supporters, advocates and auxiliaries
to the health establishment."[7] They served as fund-raisers
and lobbyists for voluntary charitable hospitals. Though
the HSA Volunteers' goals are different, their members and
political style are akin to (perhaps, an outgrowth of) the
voluntary associations. Both recruit heavily from affluent
families and spouses of community leaders. And like the
voluntary associations, the Volunteers are likely to
commit a great deal of time, they are often the "hardest
working" board members.

3. Advocates. Like the members of the preceding cate-
gory, Advocates take a systemic "public interest" view.
However, they are far more goal-oriented, approaching the
HSA with a clear vision of changes they wish to introduce.

Conceptually, any strongly held universalistic goal
fits into this category. A consumer might joint to--say--
"do something about health care costs." In practice, Advocates are most likely to promote widespread--"grass
roots"--participation and "bottoms-up" planning [with the
cost cutters in the occupationally related category (5)].
They are critical of the medical establishment and work
for sweeping reform. These are the heirs to the progressive reformers, well-educated professionals (college teachers,

lawyers, doctors) who seek to enhance democratic values while combatting an elite system. And like the progressives, they often perceive issues in highly moral terms.[8]

Advocates are least likely to ally with staff or mainstream providers. They chafe under the continual barrage of certificate-of-need reviews that dominate most HSAs. This is not systemic change but marginal regulation.

Furthermore, technical expertise does not impress them. Indeed, they are likely to respond to a statistics recitation by asking coldly for error margins and degrees of significance.

A straightforward reading of the National Health Planning Act would suggest an active role for these Advocates. The HSA task appears to involve a rethinking of the health system, advocacy for major change as much as regulatory tinkering. How else can access to health services be increased while quality is improved and costs are cut?

As one Health Systems Plan puts it: these apparently conflicting goals can be achieved if "the health care delivery system can be reshaped....Specifically, [our] aim has been to encourage a shift from a curative care system to a *community based* health promotion. . . ."[9] Generally, sweeping health system changes and community involvement has been confined to the planning documents. The time consuming grind of project reviews (usually for certificates of need) leave board members little time to consider other issues, much less a "reshaping of the health care delivery system." Most Advocates have grown discouraged and pessimistic about their HSAs. Almost everywhere, the major issues have been defined away from their concerns. (Advocates generally refer to the HSA as "they.")

4. Interest Group Champions. These representatives also have clearly articulated health system goals. But they represent the interests of a specific constituency rather than the entire public; they pursue "particularistic" rather than "universalistic" policy. While the Advocates (3) ask what this action means for the health system, Interest Group Champions wonder how it affects their constituency.

Early readings of P.L. 93-64] suggested a sort of Madisonian interest group congress: policy hashed out between representatives of relevant interests. Economic, racial, and geographic groups as well as spokesmen for those afflicted by specific illnesses took particular notice. In practice, the Champions of these interests rarely dominate HSAs (Philadelphia is the exception in this sample), but there are always some present.

In urban areas, the most visible Interest Group Champions speak for minorities and the poor. In places, they are caught in a conflict with the Advocates, though they share many attitudes. The Champion's strong sense of constituency makes them more apt to bargain for incremental benefits. For example, in several cases they voted to approve closely contested project applications from major institutions in exchange for a negotiated number of Medicaid beds. Advocates, with a more sweeping vision of equity, voted against the projects; they argued that primary care clinics, not more high-technology medicine, were needed. Advocates reminded the Interest Group Champions of their shared history of joint assaults on the large, unfeeling (in places, racist) institutions. In effect, the latter responded that the tangible benefits they had negotiated were more useful to constituents than the distant, possibly hopeless, battle they had eschewed. Charges of selling out to "golden tongued" providers were quietly exchanged. But there was no selling out. Rather, divergent visions of reform--and of the health system--were at work. The battles they fought were about what battles reformers should be fighting.

Implicit in the preceding is a very different style than analysts have generally imputed to poverty politics. The politics of conflict and the rhetoric of imminent crisis are largely absent, replaced by a sophistication rarely noted in the community action literature. Greenstone and Peterson had suggested that the Office of Economic Opportunity's Community Action Programs (CAP boards) effectively enfranchised previously shunned groups and provided them with policy making experience. Fifteen years later, many HSAs unwittingly benefit from that political socialization.[10]

Still, the lack of conflict is easy to overstate. Certainly most HSAs have seen battles, often about agency formation (who gets how many seats) or particularly traumatic issues (closing a hospital). The Champions of particular interests are most likely to be in the thick of such fights.

Geographic interests--neighborhoods, suburbs, and (especially) counties--are also championed. The Philadelphia agency, among many others, was badly entangled in the politics of geography in its early years. And rural HSAs are particularly prone to defensive areal championing.

("It may not be much, but we just prefer our hospital to
the one in the next county.")

Interest groups with a geographic perspective had been
expected to logroll HSA decisions, every area voting for
each other's projects. But the politics of the pork barrel
rests on a perception of unlimited resources (making different projects noncompetitive). It is the opposite assumption that permeates the HSAs. And many of the agencies span
too large an area to break primarily into geographic coalitions. Despite many geographic Champions who do not care
to cut costs near home, HSAs are rarely alliances of log-
rollers looking for "more."

People afflicted with specific illnesses form another
often championed interest. Representation of the mentally
ill and the handicapped is specified in the law and very
much in evidence on the boards. These representatives
often have more in common with the Volunteers (2) than
with other Interest Group Champions: they place a high
value on community service, generally respect present
health care institutions and systems and are uneasy with
conflictual politics. In general they do not pursue their
cause with an intensity that obscures other goals. Nevertheless, like all Interest Group Champions they sit on
HSA boards to advance the interest of a very specific constituency.

5. Occupational Representatives. These Representatives
speak explicitly for the organizations that employ them,
usually labor unions, insurers and large corporations. Like
the previous one, this is a category of narrow constituencies; however, from a health services perspective, they
are far more tenuous--Prudential or Aetna rather than the
poor or aged. And like the advocates they often speak
for a system-wide public interest, usually controlling
costs; however that caring is mediated by the concrete
interests that they represent. Furthermore, this is a
category of professionals: board activity forms a part of
their occupational lives.

The most delegatory approach to representation appeared
in this category. Perhaps this was predictable: large
organizations often take public policy positions; and they
have obvious mechanisms by which to hold employee-represen-
tatives to account. Union members, in particular, took
staunch, very conscious union positions when voting. In
language that almost paraphrased Edmund Burke, one respondent noted that this could be troublesome:

I am obligated to follow policy of the union. But
what if I disagree? What if new facts come to
light? I try to get it by by constituency . . . but
it's just difficult.

Similar sentiments were occasionally--far less pointed-
ly--raised by Blue Cross representatives. Still, in the
vast majority of cases, voting was said to follow from
congruent beliefs, averting any conflict between trustee
and delegatory representation: "I do vote the union
position, but I wouldn't be working for the union if I
didn't believe in its position." Private insurors or
corporate Representatives very rarely avowed a company
"position," suggesting that their occupation shaped rather
than directed their HSA perceptions. Many would deny even
representing their companies, though fellow board members
quickly (and often) demur with comments like "those guys
are serving with pay."

Unions have perhaps the most fundamentally ambiguous
perspective. Every year they must spend more bargaining
muscle for the same medical benefits. To some extent, the
cost is paid in foregone wage rises. On the other hand,
present cost control efforts--forbidding expansion, merging
services--mean fewer jobs. Different unions have responded
differently. Some work closely with the hospital industry
to preserve jobs, others fight against rising costs. In
either case, they often stake out strong positions.

Every board studied included the Representatives of
private insurance companies.[11] There is much controversy
over insurer's interests. They profit partially by invest-
ing (for three months) the money the take in; and in some
cases, fees are determined by a percentage of dollar volume. Furthermore, the problems of inflation can simply be
passed on to the consumer in higher premiums. Strong incentives, then, seem to tug insurers away from the cost containment they are so publically concerned about.

And yet, every insurer interviewed or observed in this
study fixed entirely on reducing costs--in their votes,
their speeches, their interviews there was little else but
cost control. Indeed, there was occasionally friction
between Advocates or Interest Group Champions over the
insurer's tendency to "take very element in their law and
turn it into a question of costs."

It may be that rising costs inject too much uncertainty
for their oganizations. More important, if health costs
rise faster than premiums, any advantage is lost. Insur-

ors--one spokesman claimed--are caught between inflation and competition. They need to guess at next year's medical sector inflation rate in setting their premium; but they are afraid to set it higher than their competitors.

6. Statesmen and Politicians. Some board members appear to have few referents outside the board itself. They pursue no particular health system goal or interest; they do not even seem concerned about specific health topics. Rather, they focus on the agency, its process, its politics. An HSA's founders, for example, often concern themselves with successfully establishing the HSA as an organization.

I call them Statesmen if they stand above most battles within the agency, sometimes mediating, often combatting external threats (e.g., law suits, inadequate state CON laws, a troublesome SHPDA). If, however, their energy seems directed entirely toward the battles and machinations of board politics--without outside referents or system interests, they are board politicians. This is easily the smallest of the six categories.

Both analysts and advocates have become accustomed to generalizing about "providers" and "consumers." This section has sought to unpack those designations. I have tried to show what they entail, empirically; and to suggest that it is often fatuous to use simple adjectives on such board categories.

Surely "consumers" and "providers" are motivated by systematic, often predictable, interests; and these may aggregate--sometimes, in some places--into schisms between "providers" and "consumers." But such labels (particularly the latter) press together a horde of cross-cutting interests, outlooks, styles and ambitions. Notions such as "provider dominance" and "consumer gullibility," may express no more than clashing outlooks between observers and actors. There are, to return to the respondents quoted earlier, "consumers and consumers"; the same is true--though less so--for providers, and communities of providers.

Different boards show different mixes of the categories I have described. No single one dominated across all agencies. Detroit consumers are thoroughly dominated by Organizational Representatives. In Minneapolis-St. Paul, almost all consumers are Volunteers, many of the providers are Tories. A small core of leaders in Idaho is quite similar. Philadelphia consumers are Champions and Volunteers though there are some strong Advocates seeking to redefine

the way the HSA perceives issues. Atlanta mixes, among
others, Volunteers with an increasing number of Interest
Group Champions. Every board has its share of Warm Bodies
and Warm Bodies seeking eminence, though some have more,
some fewer.

Obviously the style and tone of an HSA's politics are
shaped by its mix of types. However, in some key ways
(and with some limited exceptions) HSA outcomes vary little
across the cases studied. Precisely how and why this is
so is the topic of the following section.

ACHIEVING REPRESENTATION

This part examines some of the details of representing
consumers--how they are selected, assigned to committees,
put to tasks, and trained. Such details shape the success
(and failure) of representation. Ultimately the major
argument presented here is that the proponents of repre-
sentation--as well as the law--have been overly diffuse in
their efforts. There is, from a reformer's perspective,
many good impulses in the National Health Planning Act;
but some are better than others. And they are not always
completely compatible.

Selecting the Board

The National Health Planning Act never specified how
representatives should be selected. The agencies were left
to devise their own processes. There was far less variation than predicted, but some clear patterns emerge.

1. *Elections.* I had predicted that elections along the
school board model would result in low turnout and unsuccessful representation. As it happens, none of the
HSAs conducts direct elections.

However, Philadelphia holds elections through the mail.
Despite a cumbersome (very expensive) process, about 30,000
"HSA members"--essentially citizens who have registered--
cast votes in the last election (run by the American Arbitration Association, rather than the agency). The election
is indirect, candidates run for SACs, SACs vote members to
the governing board. Consequently, my hypotheses could
not be examined--SAC attendance was low ("50 percent at

best," said one respondent) but this is a problem endemic to SACs, aggravated by uncertain roles and cramped resources.

Indirect elections can have a great deal in common with selection by organizations--the board members tend to be experienced and competent in organizational politics and have clear constituencies, with well defined (i.e., local, geographic) interests. These observations hold, however, only where SACs are relatively vital (those in Philadelphia are--for all their problems--the most active of the ones in this sample); they must, for example, have functions other than merely selecting members to the governing board.

2. *Self-selection*. This has been one of the poorest selection modes. Often citizens clip an application and submit it with little idea of what board membership entails; occasionally individuals who have not even expressed interest are "drafted"--asked to fill out applications so they can be selected. Typically, HSA selection committees pore over applications searching for demographic types (e.g., poverty representatives) or brainstorm about community notables who might be induced to serve. As I suggested earlier, neither tends to make effective board members.*

Many of the criticisms that have been made of merely descriptive representation--seating board members only

------

* In determining "effectiveness" of individual board members I scaled three items:

Representation--Each respondent was asked to name the board members they thought were most effective. (They were urged to consider representatives with varying viewpoints.) Respondents named by two people (whether consumer, provider, or staff) received one point, those named by 30 percent or those questioned received 2.

Knowledge--Representatives familiar with major local HSA issues received +1, those unfamiliar with them received -1.

Participation--Representatives who participated at meetings received +1, those that dominated a meeting (e.g., changing a vote with a dramatic speech) received +2. Those who never participated were scored 0. Those who were regularly absent received -1. +2 is added to all scores so that they can range from 0 to +7.

The following categories were constructed:

    0-3 Ineffective
    4-5 Effective
    6-7 Very Effective

because they "fit" in the demographic criteria--are borne out in agencies that recruit in this fashion. A harassed staff member sarcastically illustrated the problem in a late night meeting: "Now if only we can find a black, Roman Catholic, 65-year-old nun, we'll have representation."

The revision of the health planning law (P.L. 96-79) limits self-selecting HSAs. Only 50 percent of the board can be selected in this fashion. Though the change was made to restrict exclusionary boards, it is an important one for limiting ineffective board members. The danger, of course, is that mainly consumers will continue to be self-selected while providers are all chosen by their interest groups.

3. *Selection By Organized Interests*. Elsewhere in this volume I argue that representatives be selected by organized interests. An empirical analysis by TARP, Inc. (May 1979) reached the same conclusion. Selection by (and association with) organized health care interests is the best predictor of effective consumer representation in this sample as well. The following characteristics typify the effective respondents (futhermore, they were also the answers most commonly given to the question, "what typifies effective board members?"):

a. An active interest. A minimal criteria, given the time demands.

b. Experience in political and organizational pro-cesses. HSA processes are complicated, easily overwhelming; and in three of the six cases, a majority of respondents spoke in terms of extensive politicking, bargaining, and outside political contacts. Political neophytes are often bewildered.

c. A clear sense of purpose (generally for Advocates).

d. A clear sense of constituency.

These last (but especially d) tend to give board members a clear sense of legitimacy in the often perplexing world of technical planning. Repeatedly--and in every site--I was told that "the good representative is the one that isn't afraid to ask the dumb question." Representatives who know precisely why they are on the board are more likely to ask that question than to be swept along.

Many representatives evinced the preceding attributes. However, selection by organized health interests is the most typical screen for them.

There is one exceptional type, often "effective," often demonstrating the characteristics listed here, that are not associated with this, or any other, selection mode:

the Volunteers. Yet they, too, generally showed political and organizational experience. They were not usually selected by organizations, but were almost always closely affiliated with them.

It is often suggested that representatives with clear (and organized) constituencies would fracture the boards and undermine the HSA process. This view is incorrect, partly because of the inexorable nature of that process. For consumers, there is a tremendously centripetal force operating within HSAs. Regardless of initial interests, they are flooded with new terms, new concepts and plain work. It all carries a strong socializing effect. To become a board member with some clout, the new terms have to be learned, the concepts understood, the work done. Consumer representatives are coopted--not by providers-- but by the agency itself. Far from fracturing the HSA, clear constituencies help representatives keep their bear- ings--their sense of purpose--in all the details.

I had anticipated that an organization's resources and the necessity to report to it would help shape effective representation. In the sites I visited, neither was rele- vant.

4. *Local Government.* Local government officials vary enormously in their effectiveness. The category includes some of the strongest and the weakest representatives in this sample. The key may be of interest: public officials are prime candidates for being "drafted" onto the boards; they are often Eminents. Unless an official cares about health care and HSA issues, he or she will treat the agency as just another commission of which to be a member. On two of the HSAs, respondents spoke very critically of public officials on the board. One case that particularly rankled was triggered when a public official, making a rare appearance at a tumultuous meeting, addressed the HSA by the wrong name ("Fellow Health Service Commission mem- bers").

Furthermore, placing public officials on boards rarely serves a liaison function between local government and the HSA, as some commentators had expected. The interests of a single official are often distinct from local (and almost always from state) government interests.

Local officials can also *select* board members (Idaho, Minneapolis/St. Paul, Chicago); however, it is difficult to see consistent patterns across the sites in this model. It may be that the effectiveness of the board will be as good as the government that selects it. In any case, this form

of selection will not, alone, establish the legitimacy of
HSAs as a governmental unit. Idaho illustrates the point
dramatically. Using public elected officials to select
the board (they appoint to the SAC which elects the governing board) has done nothing to tame an angry, hostile,
anti-regulatory political environment that includes the
state legislature and (at least till very recently) the
SHPDA.

And yet, as the overturns and rebuffs described below
will illustrate, finding a legitimate place in the local
process is crucial for HSAs. In this sample, only Minne-
apolis/St. Paul has not had difficulties with the political
system about it. This is a consequence, not of their
selection scheme but the agency's organizational chart--it
answers directly to a local governmental authority, the
Metropolitan Council (in fact, the latter--rather than the
HSA itself--received designation at the inception of P.L.
93-641). Ironically, of the six agencies examined, DHHS
has been most critical of intergovernmental relationships
in this case.

Participation and Representation

The public mostly doesn't give a damn. A perfect
illustration is a series of public hearings held by
the North Central Georgia [Atlanta] HSA [regarding]
the agency's . . . Health Systems Plan.
Twenty-eight people showed up at the four hearings.
And in one case all four who came were members of
the HSA board; in other words, not a single ordi-
nary citizen attended. (Richard Mathews, Atlanta
Journal. Feb. 19, 1980)

Everywhere, similar sentiments are expressed. Not a
single respondent indicated that public participation was
"very high"; not a single site showed more than sporadic
twitchings of public concern over specific projects. But
all this merely underscores the difference--emphasized
elsewhere in this volume--between participation and representation. What is most distinctive about HSAs is that
they are directed, not by professional planners, but by
representative boards whose function it is to speak for
the public. The striking news in the Journal article, cited
above, is not that no one in Griffin came to speak out
about the "bureaucratically dull" but "incredibly important"

plans; rather, it is what is taken for granted--the board
members were there. When the concentrated provider interests do not come, and consumer representative do--the
best odds in political and organizational theory are being
beaten.

Participation by the general citizenry is largely an
anachronistic ideal; representation, difficult in its own
right, a modern substitute. Neither the frustration often
voiced regarding the former, nor its occasional successes
(*vide* Checkoway and the western Massachusetts HSA) should
obscure the more relevant, more important efforts of
citizen representatives to organize HSAs. (In many cases,
it was very much the board members--and especially the
consumers--that put the agency together.)

In contrast, almost every respondent dismissed local
"public participation" as a show, choreographed by providers submitting projects: "in meeting after meeting, out
come the carefully done up dog and pony shows." Throughout this sample, empirical observation reflects political
theory in suggesting the importance of representation over
participation.

This is not to denigrate the public participation provisions in P.L. 96-79. There certainly have been some
instances of communities exploding with support or criticism over a specific policy: the outpouring of support
from Atlanta's black community over a proposal by Southwest
Community Hospital, for example, genuinely affected many
local board members. Similarly, Operation PUSH organized
the intense sentiments of a poor neighborhood in Detroit
over the closing of Martin Place West Hospital.

It is important for such genuine community sentiments
to be heard. And the National Health Planning Act's
participatory provisions (e.g., open publicized hearings)
present them with an important forum. But reformers are
too easily distracted from the central, institutional
issue: effective, consumer-dominated agencies.

The Planning Act promises consumer majorities. Trans-
lating them into a force that can direct HSAs takes tremendous effort. Consumers must be selected in a fashion
that is likely to recruit competent and interested board
members; they have to be prepared--though the appropriate
mix of educational tools is an open question; and they
must fashion an agency process that facilitates rather than
impedes consumer contributions. In short, the detailed
implementation of consumer representation is a painstaking,
complex process. But it makes all the difference to con-

sumer success. Reforms such as open meetings, well attended forums, many sub-area councils, media attention, color brochures, monthly newsletters, etc., all are secondary.

Advocates of consumer representation can easily get lost in long lists of good reformist things that HSAs do. But they can all distract from the central task: institutionalizing consumer representation within the agency. Those citizens of Griffin may come to forums or (as is more likely) not; the crucial question is how well their representatives are learning to direct the HSA in their name.

The Other Side of "Reform"

The cautions about overestimating participation can be cast more emphatically. Broad participation is not merely an ideal--often feigned, sporadically attained--that is likely to distract reformers. It can more directly undermine their reforms. Task forces illustrate one opportunity.

Task forces have tremendous potential for spreading participation and tapping community sentiment. And governing boards rarely hae the time or the capacity for such detailed work. Task forces, then, are necessary and laudable. But a problem: tremendous energy and attention is being (or ought to be) devoted to establishing effective recruitment procedures, training, and organization of governing boards. Task forces are blithely oblivious to such troubles: they are recruited--certainly on these HSAs--by a very small number of agency members, usually staff. They have not been trained in or socialized into the politics and processes of the HSA. They are usually unaware of issues that might be raging in the agency. As a consequence they are reliant on their staff for anything more than their own sentiments and/or expertise.

This is not meant to denigrate task forces, *per se*. On the contrary, they are an integral part of any HSA. They carry tremendous potential for tapping both expert and public opinion. Surely a panel of physician experts, to cite one case I saw, is essential to meaninful rules about cardiac catheterization. Rather, the point here is that task forces must be established with careful regard to agency processes. They ought to exist within the framework of a well-functioning governing board, dominated by consumers; not threaten it. And they can be a threat: that representative board can be tilted or circumvented by the judicious use of task forces. This is a "reform" that merits careful attention by consumers.

Naturally, task forces report to larger committees, but to think that they will scrutinize the results is to ignore the organizational realities of most (though not all) the HSAs. The details of weeks, often months, of work are usually reviewed only superficially by board committees already loaded down with their own work. Task force recommendations can pass swiftly into review criteria (for example). By the time they are applied, they are an implicit part of the process and difficult to change.

Committees

All HSA committees--like the governing boards themselves-- must reflect the community's mix of demographic character- istics.* One, completely unanticipated, consequence par- allels the dynamic just described on taks forces--the con- centration of authority within the HSAs. Selecting the "proper" mix of demographic types can be extremely complex. In one agency, board members can alter a slate (selected in large part by a staff member) of candidates for the powerful executive committee only by threading additional names into 1 of 30 categories (income x county x race).

In another agency, the nominating committee simply chooses an executive committee, without even a comment from the governing board; respondents frankly reported that this was a vestige of the original core of board members who wished to retain control of the agency that they had organized.

In a third HSA, one officer told me bluntly that his control over committee appointments was used to make sure the "toughest members" of the board were on the committee that does reviews. In two other sites, respondents won- dered aloud whether the staff role in committee selection was excessive, and whether it biased the committees toward the staff's goals.

Regardless of whether it is staff, officers, or govern-

---

* How the planning amendments will alter the following ob- servations--if at all--is not clear. Note, however, that all observations reported here precede their implementa- tion.

ing board cliques, the often intricate representational criteria for HSA committees places the task of selecting those committees in a small number of hands. Often it is treated as just another task; but it is always at least an opportunity to bias the organization and its process.

Aids

Consumer representatives had a clear, surprising answer to questions about education of board members: they were *for* it, of course. But not one respondent thought they had been much affected by their educational sessions: few thought that their agency provided effective ones; and it was not generally considered a major priority. (There were, interestingly, many scattered references to other HSAs and what good educational processes they were reputed to have; but even following some of those citations to the agencies reputed to have the good processes did not produce a different set of responses.

Rather, consumers most often said they went to staff with technical questions or--more generally--HSA problems. Perhaps the most useful "orientation session" in this sample was the board member who simply invited every member of the staff to lunch, one at a time. Naturally this is unusual, not often replicable; but it makes the crucial point: the most important consumer aid is an accessible, willing staff. For consumers, staff is a capable, full time resource, balancing potentially imbalanced political markets. Developing a close, working relationship is imperative.

Note that some of the consumer categories are more likely to clash with staff members than others. If Advocates have goals that clash with the staff's, then orientations, technical discussions--even lunch--are not likely to be much use.

Accountability

The major unfulfilled expectation of the planning act is the failure of providers to achieve dominance. Other papers in this volume describe the expectation of imbalance at some length. Note that the actual dynamics of imbalance and concentrated stakes have not been vitiated, not even-- necessarily--overcome in P.L. 96-79. Rather, the concentrated interest of professional planning staffs was underestimated. In almost every case, they have shown a

tenacious commitment to rationalization, planning and
cost control that was quite unforeseen. In doing so,
they have often balanced the concentrated stakes of provider representatives.

The intensity of the staff's interest is a result,
not only of their training or their outlook, but of the
accountability structured into the law. There was meant
to be a dynamic tension in Rational Health Planning--
Washington overseeing community input. And certainly the
tension exists. In Atlanta, three-fourths of the respondents had intensely negative views about DHHS; and the
executive director testified at the hearings sponsored by
the National Academy of Sciences that "to be considered
a federal agency is an invitation to failure." In Detroit
HSA critics were told: "it is either us or a Federal
czar." In Idaho, the same sentiment was echoed by every
respondent; and the HSA stationery pointedly proclaims
"the health planning by Idaho for Idaho." And yet, the
behavior of the agency--and particularly its professionals--
is fundamentally shaped by the federal perspective. When
Idaho HSA officials testified on their state's certificate-
of-need law, they were blasted for simply parroting the
perspective of the federal government that they were generally so critical of in their interviews.

The tension between Washington and the community remains
strikingly in evidence. But there is no synthesis of
the polar interests and visions. Local and federal interests are not complementary so much as clashing. Despite
all efforts, to paraphrase Rudolf Klein, this circle
obstinately refuses to be squared. And in P.L. 96-79, it
is accountability to Washington that emerges triumphant.
DHHS monitors the agencies; their funding is at stake. No
other interest or actor in the HSA environment can match
the lever at DHHS' disposal--organizational survival. Regardless of all the comments to the contrary, that fact
affects the outlook of every staffer that I talked to; it
affects the outlook of every board member that gets socialized into the HSA process; it fundamentally shapes the HSAs.

Process and Role

In every HSA, the word heard most often is "process": the
proudest accomplishment of the early HSA years is invariably
"setting up a good process"; a problem is being dealt with
if it is "in process"; it has them licked if "there is no

process to deal with it." The constant repetition points to a major issue: establishing these governmental structures--writing bylaws, recruiting staff and governing board, deciding which committee ought to do what, when--has all consumed tremendous time. It is, in fact, the accomplishment that a majority of HSA leaders say they are most proud of. And it is a set of issues that still snares five out of six of these agencies. Idaho is rewriting its bylaws, committees in Philadelphia are trying to determine their tasks and--more important--their relationships, likewise the committees in Atlanta and Detroit have been trying to determine the most appropriate way for board to interact with staff. More examples are easily come by.

These efforts at setting a process straight can be conceived of as ways of getting the governing board to "mesh"--to interact in a significant fashion, articulate mutual underlying perspectives and perceive the same agency goals and problems. To put it negatively, an agency where board members do not know each other's names--or HSA tasks--is not "meshing." The governing board is probably not genuinely governing so much as voting on things that are brought before it.

The huge size of HSA governing boards significantly retards this process. The average board has 44 members, they range up to 137. These are simply too big to interact significantly. In fact, most agency control is usually passed to the executive committee (Philadelphia is the exception in this sample)--the governing board is too large, too unwieldy, and meets too infrequently to establish a process that "meshes." The consumer success and knowledge (referred to at the start of this essay) is largely limited to executive committees--or, in some cases, parts of them.

A major question, is then: Why not encourage smaller, governing boards comprised of the more articulate, interested, involved? Save the massive governing board membership their few annual trips downtown. Any committee too large to pursue a reasonable conversation is too large to reasonably govern an agency.

Paring down the governing board would mean finding one poverty representative (rather than the half dozen that so many agencies are having so much trouble finding). That one representative would have a tremendously enhanced role, sitting around a small table rather than at the distant reaches of a huge one. And if competition for the one spot developed, the bulk of democratic theorizing suggests that it would enhance accountability and representation; one representative--in a small group--is more easily held to account than six lost in a crowd of sixty.*

The objection, of course, is workload. No one--when off the record--expects the huge governing board to actually govern. Rather it forms a "bullpen" of surplus labor. Consumers are dolloped out, to each HSA function, legitimating whatever is being done. They work assiduously, learn tremendous amounts; and usually remain ignorant of how the agency they govern fits together (until perhaps they sit on an executive committee or, in some places, the still smaller board of officers).

And yet, it might be an advantage if--with fewer numbers--HSAs could not accomplish all that work. It might force a reconsideration of what it is consumers do. They seek to dominate the HSAs; they are set to a huge number of tasks and work, many of them, extraordinarily hard at it: to what purpose?

The question, finally, is one that is rarely addressed: consumers for what? Or put still another way, what is the consumer role?

Surely something is not right when volunteers must spend up to 20 hours a week in order to contribute. Surely consumers were expected, somehow, to oversee more and do less.

The issue is easy for corporate boards--if profit levels are unacceptable, action may be necessary: clear criteria, relatively clear range of responses.

And boards of hospitals, or community representatives in England, work with a similarly clear role: Mediate between consumers of a service and its providers. HSAs, of course, deliver no such services; consumer representatives have no such obvious direction.

The HSA consumer role is, I shall argue in the next section, a problem that is being resolved--though not by conscious choice. An extraordinary program has been developed; extraordinary combinations of people--Blue Cross presidents and poverty lawyers--have begun a dialogue

---

*Note incidentally that small size is only one element that would facilitate HSA "meshing"; a greater time frame for review with its concomittant bargaining would be another important one.

over the shape of local health systems. I shall suggest,
however, that HSA "process" and its dominant activity makes
such dialogues increasingly less central to the HSAs.

PROJECT REVIEW AND THE INEXORABLE PROCESS OF PROCESS

The dominant HSA activity is "project review," the matching
of capital expenditures proposals with its health systems
plan. The procedure is roughly (and vastly simplified)
this: a hospital files a project (say 10 new acute care
beds). A committee of the HSA investigates the "need"
for that project. Staff members to that committee analyze
it, making either a formal recommendation or limiting
their analyses to ostensibly neutral "findings of fact."
The crux of the issue lies in the criteria relevant to
the proposed project:* for example, how many similar beds
are there within 30 minutes travel time? how many are there
in the county? does the hospital have the resources for
the project? are there less costly alternatives? By checking the proposed project with the--often relatively intri-
cate--criteria, the committee can determine whether there
is "need" (thus warranting a certificate of need). The
committee (sometimes a subarea council) sends its recommendation to the major deliberative body. That body varies
among HSAs--often it is the executive committee, occasionally the governing board as a whole. After another round
of presentations by the applicant and the staff, the
executive committee or governing board decides whether or
not to uphold the committee's finding. In most places, the
time limits of certificate-of-need laws preclude remanding
an item to the committee for further study. A case must
be introduced, deliberated, and disposed of at one meeting.
    Project review generally dominates HSAs. It is the
major focus of media attention, lobbying, politics, and late
night meetings. In many places, plan implementation--the
shaping of the health system's future--means little more
than accepting or denying hospital proposals. Almost all
providers and most consumers interviewed talked in project
terms. There were, to be sure, staff and occasional Advocates pointing to many other far less visible functions.

---

* The criteria are most often developed by task forces and
submitted to the governing board in the process described
in the section entitled "Achieving Representation."

However, the bulk of the discussion for every category of respondent was about project review. "The rest is baloney" according to more than one respondent.

A majority of the respondents also spoke of the futility of cost cutting in this fashion. Their major criticisms were:

1. Certificate of need--which varies significantly from state to state[13]--affects hospital investment but not doctors' offices.

2. In most places, it does nothing about what most (respondents) see as the real culprit behind rising costs--current reimbursement patterns [an opinion ironically echoed by P.L. 96-79, itself, sec. 1502(b)(1)].

3. The federal projects that HSAs review and comment on are still more frustrating. As they are already budgeted, these funds will be used, if not on the project being reviewed, then for some other. Vladeck had suggested that HSAs would be loathe to turn down tangible benefits for something as distant as health care cost savings;[11] the poignancy of federal fund reviews is that even when board members are willing to seek cost control, they are rebuffed with the knowledge that the federal spigot cannot be slowed, but merely shunted elsewhere. (It is a knowledge that particularly rankles conservative board members who are ill-disposed to the federal projects, such as half-way houses and clinics, that are generally reviewed.)

4. Respondents often noted the reactive nature of present project review--rather than determining what is needed and seeking to accomplish it, HSAs generally determine what is needed, then process applications to see if they--more or less--fit. The details, the work flow, the initiative are all set by the applicant institutions, not by the health care planners.

5. A small number of respondents criticize the whole idea of certificate of need on equity grounds--"If I've got my linear accelerator, you probably won't get yours, even if you have a more sensible place for it."

6. The preceding were often noted, but ultimately peripheral. A more fundamental problem undermines HSAs and their cost containment efforts: the difficult struggle for agency legitimacy. HSAs are structured on a quasi-corporatist principle. The key to corporatist decision-making is that representatives have the final say--they speak for both their constituency and the government. The compromise that they hash out is expected to become policy.

The HSA process forms almost the reverse case. The agencies
constantly fight to preserve their legitimacy as decision-
makers in a system that appears to barely notice their
existence. The point is illustrated dramatically by the
six cases in my sample.

> In Idaho, the HSA turned down a nursing home
> (Blaine Home) application. It was only the
> agency's second refusal and was considered a
> difficult step for a relatively young organiza-
> tion in a hotly antiregulatory political environ-
> ment. But as with their previous rejection, IHSA
> was overruled on the state level. The director of
> the Department of Health and Welfare, in announc-
> ing the overrule, simply did not address the cause
> of IHSA rejection (i.e., there were less expen-
> sive alternatives available to the applicant).*

> In Philadelphia, two hospitals that were denied
> CAT scanners simply purchased them nonetheless.
> Blue Cross refused to reimburse the hospitals for
> interest, depreciation and operation expenses
> (31-32 percent of the patients were Blue Cross
> subscribers). However, spokesmen for a major
> private insurer suggested that if the private
> companies were to take action, they would be
> liable for antitrust. "The hospital will simply
> shift the costs to the private insurors."*

> In Detroit, the University of Michigan applied for
> a $251 million project, replacing the University
> of Michigan building. The HSA thought the plan
> extravagant and sought to reduce it by roughly
> $50 million and 48 beds. (The area is said to have
> 3,400 excess beds.) HSA representatives were so
> infuriated by the hospital's "complete unwilling-
> ness to even acknowledge" them that the executive
> council voted *unanimously* to reject the proposal
> (a most unusual outcome, noted one respondent).
> They were more infuriated still when the State CON
> agency approved the project at $244 million--
> without consulting the HSA.

------

*In these cases, CON laws were not yet in place and re-
views were done on the basis of Sec. 1122 of the Social
Security Act.

In Atlanta, two psychiatric hospitals were reviewed simultaneously (batched)--after tremendous
strife, one was approved, one rejected. The
state agency (SHPDA) simply approved both.

Springfield--at the time of my site visit--had
not turned any projects down.

Only Minneapolis had not had to contend with this
issue of its standing as an agency.

In each case, the HSA argued that "the integrity of the
planning process is at stake." In each case, their own
legitimacy was undermined--not by a professional decision
overruling the "amateurs" but by political decisions that
undercut very difficult--often painful--decisions by the
HSA board members.

   7. Finally, and more than anything else, respondents--
consumer staff and even providers--commented on the crush-
ing grind of the process. At public hearings sponsored by
the National Academy of Sciences in March 1980, one person
testified that a board member had stacked his HSA documents
till they stood taller than he, even when he stood on his
desk. That image, an overwhelming deluge of materials,
procedures, criteria--just plain "process"--is the most
basic and overwhelming fact of board membership. Advocacy
and fights and issues come and go, but the deluge of material to be digested and acted on--generally with a strict
(CON imposed) time limit and a welter of regulations and
procedures to conform to--does not abate.

   An important distinction exists on most HSAs between
what can be termed "regulatory" and "political" orientations. The former is typified by the impartial application of pre-formulated rules (e.g., only 4 beds/1,000 in
each county); if there are more, no new beds regardless
of the circumstance. This is the classic bureaucratic-
regulatory approach. It clashes with a more political
vision that decides on a case by case basis. The political
decisions, of course, are often criticized for being an
application of irrelevant criteria.

   Both types of decision-maker are apparent--to more or
less a degree--on every HSA. Often, different parts of
the agency typify the different modes. In Atlanta, for
example, the project review committee staunchly follows
the established criteria when reviewing a project; the
executive committee, on the other hand, is apt to inject

other considerations--the reputation of the hospital in question, for example. The friction between the two committees is generally thought to be the major line of conflict among board members, subsuming even provider-consumer conflict. In Philadelphia, staff and some consumers (Volunteers, Organizational Representatives) embody the regulatory ethic and generally stand opposed to (institutional) provider representatives showing solidarity with the applicant, city representatives seeking money for Philadelphia, and representatives of the poor seeking more services (Interest Group Champions). In every site, at least some respondents argued that merely "political" decision-making is unsophisticated, that it undermines any possibility of rationalizing health services and cutting costs. It is often considered "selling out" to the providers.

And yet, why have a governing board to simply apply (often subtly biased) criteria--generally fashioned by the staff and approved by the board long ago? Why, as three respondents in Atlanta asked, "do they need con-sumers if they could just plug in a computer [to] check the statistics and see if they fit?" Underlying their question is the fact that--unlike bureaucracies--governing boards are biased, against the impartial application of preformulated rules.

Consequently, victories for the regulatory approach require--in many agencies--overcoming the natural bias of this organizational form. It often takes extraordinary energy, for the pressure is enormous. It involves--to take an incident I witnessed in three cases--board members so fixed on a series of abstract criteria that they can dismiss a provider dramatically announcing how many people will die if they say "no" to his application. (Followed, generally, by one of the patients who would have been dead if not for a similar project.)

In short, it takes confidence, knowledge, often courage, to turn down a project. But again, the major questions: why have we launched so massive a program of consumer representation, only to transform citizen representatives into amateur bureaucrats, striving to hold down costs through a project review system that undermines their almost every attempt to do so?

The fundamental question about consumer representation is not "What can we do to make them more effective?" but rather, "Have we set them to the right task?" Is this what we really want the consumer representatives to be doing?

The law itself is studded with innovative possibilities:
deinstitutionalization of mental patients, increased use
of physician extenders, HMOs, alternate reimbursement
systems, access for poor and rural populations, quality
of care. HSAs sound like they are intended as shapers
of the local health systems of the future.

The point is not that HSAs never address such issues--
many do; rather, the consumers--burdened by project re-
view--pay peripheral attention to them. Rather than
"sitting down and thinking about the kind of system [the]
community ought to have," they process review applications.
Rather than considering alternative values they apply criteria. They are more questions of computation than of
judgment.

The argument of this section is simple: an extraordinary resource has been developed, and is being wasted.
A large number of the respondents appreciated the ultimate
futility of their struggle to regulate costs. Consumer
representatives are doing well, they are not doing much
good.

REFERENCES

1. "Repeal of Health Planning Act Urged." *American Medical News* 22:15, August 3/10, 1979.

2. Florida Public Health Review Project. Sponsored by the College of Social and Behavioral Sciences, University of South Florida, Tampa, July 6-7, 1977.

3. Wayne Clarke, *Placebo or Cure? State and Local Health Planning Agencies in the South.* Southern Governmental Monitoring Project, Southern Regional Council, Atlanta, 1977.

4. See Larry Brown, "Structural Issues in Health Planning," elsewhere in this volume, for an analysis of competing HSA tasks.

5. See reference 1.

6. See Harvey Sapolsky, "Bottoms Up Is Upside Down," elsewhere in this volume.

7. Elena Padilla, "Community Participation in Health Affairs," in Arthur Levin (ed.), *Health Services: The Local Perspective.* Proceedings of the Academy of Political Science, Vol. 32, No. 3, New York, 1977.

8. See Grant McConnell, *Private Power and American Democracy* (Vintage Books, New York, 1966), for a discussion of contemporary American politics and its links to the Progressive era.

9. The Comprehensive Health Planning Council of Southeast Michigan. *Health Systems Plan*, Detroit, 1979, p. IV-4.

10. J. David Greenstone and Paul Peterson. *Race and Authority in Urban Politics: Community Participation and the War on Poverty*. University of Chicago Press, Chicago, 1973.

11. I am grateful to Bruce Vladeck for his instructive comments on this topic.

12. Barry Checkoway, "Consumerism in Health Planning," elsewhere in this volume.

13. See in particular, Donald Cohodes, "Interstate Variation in Certificate of Need Programs. A Review and Prospectus," elsewhere in this volume.